EQUUS

How We Misunderstand the Nature of the Horse-Human Relationship—Plus, Brave New Ideas for the Future

Trafalgar Square
North Pomfret, Vermont

Francesco De Giorgio &
José De Giorgio-Schoorl

First published in the United States of America in 2016 by
Trafalgar Square Books
North Pomfret, Vermont 05053

Originally published in the Italian language as *Comprendere il cavallo: per migliorare il rapporto con lui.* Authors: Francesco De Giorgio and José De Giorgio-Schoorl

(www.giunti.it)

English translation by Francesco De Giorgio and José De Giorgio-Schoorl

Trafalgar Square Books encourages the use of approved safety helmets in all equestrian sports and activities.

Library of Congress Control Number: 2016960008
ISBN: 978-1-57076-798-2

Photos courtesy of Learning Animals | Institute for Zooanthropology
Cover image by James Ward, *A Cossack Horse in a Landscape,* 1820s, Berger Collection at the Denver Art Museum (Photo courtesy of the Denver Art Museum)

Book design by Lauryl Eddlemon
Cover design by RM Didier
Typefaces: DIN, Frutiger
Printed in Canada
10 9 8 7 6 5 4 3 2 1

This book is dedicated to our
lifetime equine companions:

Pioggia, Marea, Ninfa, Onda,
Topazio, Fulmine, Falò, Sparta

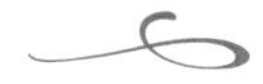

Contents

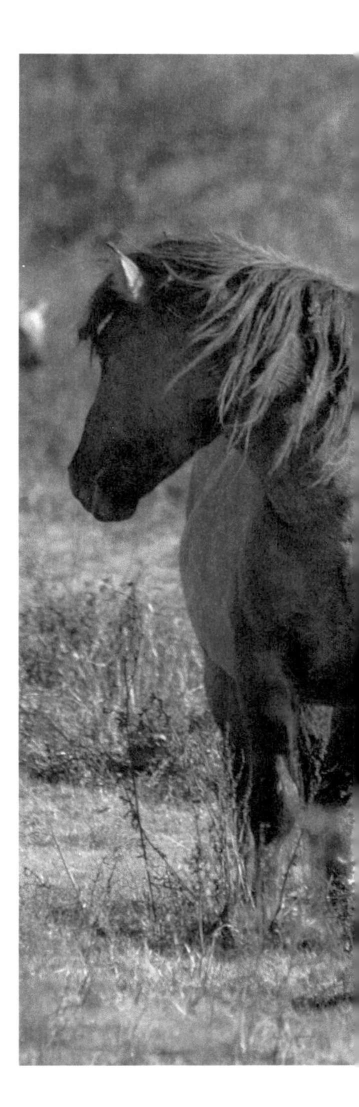

Note to the Reader

There exists an "Other" horse, too often invisible. It's the cognitive horse, and this book will take you along a path to discover where he is hiding.

It is a journey that will enable you to look at the horse from a different perspective, from the socio-cognitive point of view, which allows you to gain a better understanding, as well as a more profound awareness of the horse's world of perception. These are beneficial for the well-being of the horse, as well as for a sound, reciprocal relationship between horses and human beings.

The ideas proposed in this book are based on a model developed by Dr. Francesco De Giorgio called *Socio-Cognitive Learning* (the *SCL* model) that has its roots in a cognitive-constructivist framework in which horses, dogs, and animals in general, find their own way of dialogue with the world, creating subjective realities through cognitive learning, emancipating themselves from training and conditioning, and therefore preserving or recovering their innate cognitive heritage. The model is translated by José De Giorgio-Schoorl for human animals in their personal and professional paths of growth, in their interaction with human and non-human animals, and in general in their own dialogue with the world. This socio-cognitive model is applied in several countries in professional areas of work in the fields of animal ethics, animal welfare, animal protection, human/nonhuman interaction, human education, and academic innovation. The SCL model is taught at Learning Animals, the international institute of animal studies, ethics, and zooanthropology (www.learninganimals.com).

What Else You'll Find

Throughout the book, you will also read short stories, tales, adventures, and imaginings excerpted from the personal day-to-day life of Francesco De Giorgio; his life choices that defined him and guided him since he was a young boy—a life of cognition, emotion, and relationships in his coexistence with other animals, and today in particular with his wife José, co-author of this book, and the animals that live with them.

These life experiences are crucial to understanding the concepts that sustain and support the content of this book, but also to understanding the origin of it all, the meaning, the values, and the knowledge that make the journey these authors are undertaking—and that which they share with all those people interested in their key message, their teachings, and their mission—so immensely strong.

Zooanthropology brings a cultural movement, part of the human-animal studies, that allows a rediscovering and studying of relationships between human and other animals from an understanding and perspective that has been unthinkable until now. Thanks to the continuous contributions of Francesco and José to academics while translating their ideas into daily practice, this area of study is fascinating countries throughout the world. A thorough understanding of this field requires, however, that the human step away from the center of attention in the human-animal relationship dynamic, and from there, immerse himself in the exchange and dialogue, from a reciprocal level of understanding—animal among animals.

A Helpful Glossary

As you read, you may come upon some terms little used in equestrian literature. Here, in brief, is what Francesco and José mean when they use certain words in explaining their research, their position, and their theories:

Affiliative: behavior that promotes group cohesion (friendly/positive gestures).

Agonistic: associated with conflict.

Automatisms: spontaneous reactions or behaviors.

Complementarity: working well together.

Consolatory: the act of consoling and part of the category of affiliative behaviors.

Deterministic: an approach that proposes that all behavior is caused by precedents and is thus predictable.

Dialogical: relating to, or characterized by dialogue.

Elaborate/elaborating/elaboration: to work out carefully or minutely.

Hierarchical focus: tendency to focus on order of rank.

Hybridization: mixing experiences; sharing an experience being inspired by another's perception and point of view.

Limbic system: comprised of brain structures that are involved in emotions. These structures include the amygdala, hippocampus, and thalamus.

Proprioception: sensory information that contributes to one's sense of body position and movement.

Reductionist: the practice of simplifying a complex idea, issue, and condition.

Speciesism/anti-speciesism: speciesism involves the assignment of different values, rights, or special consideration to individuals solely on the basis of their species membership; anti-speciesism rejects the animal of the species as being a sentient being, and uses this as an argument for disregarding its interests and its life.

Zooanthropology: see sidebar on p. 16.

Introduction

This book is not a manual. There are plenty of manuals about horses and about the way they are used, their training and conditioning.

Equus Lost? is dedicated to horses as sentient and socio-cognitive living beings, to their world of perception, their acquisition of knowledge, their understanding of the environment, and their social abilities toward each other and toward humans.

This focus is necessary, because until now, following conventional paradigms, horse behavior has been mostly explained in the context of behaviorism and classic ethology (the scientific and objective study of animal behavior). These interpretations have marked the way we look at horses and how we explain their behavior, both in coexistence with each other and in their relationship with human beings.

In daily life, many things—wrongly taken for granted—create the many misunderstandings that horses encounter daily with people all over the world, and vice versa.

The way horses live in the social context, how they learn from it, and how they gather information from these surroundings and interactions, are still being thoroughly devalued, which causes a lack of proper understanding about their well-being.

There needs to be a better understanding of the horse from a cognitive point of view in order to offer knowledge and insight that will improve horses' well-being and allow for more transparency in the horse-human relationship.

This book encourages the reader to put aside many beliefs nurtured by the vast heredity of horse culture because they limit your perception despite the best of intentions. It invites you to look at known images from a different point of view, guiding toward a different perception to see horses' individual and social behavior, their emotional and affiliated needs, their social mind, and their social relationship with man. This perception will allow you to expand your horizons and develop a consciousness that will show you can learn to become aware of their world and their dialogue with those around them.

▶ *There is a world to explore in the socio-cognitive ability of the horse that will change the current anthropocentric view of the horse-human relationship. Look, it is there, just beyond the horizon.*

Learning how to look at things differently allows for the development of a new understanding. More importantly, it introduces horse cognition into your daily practice with horses and encourages further research developments and raises philosophical questions.

Equus Lost? takes the reader into a dimension where relationships are free of any tension—no leadership, dominance, or other controlling assumptions. It is a dimension based on the knowledge of the socially balanced mind of the cognitive horse that is curious and driven by his own inner motivation to explore and understand the world around him, including his relationship with humans. Reading the book means going on a journey of awareness of the animal mind, emotions, and intentions.

It introduces the concept of equine *zooanthropology* and the principles of the cognitive-zooanthropological model, which explains the elements and fundamentals in the development of a reciprocal horse-human relationship, and how to recognize and take into account the horse's socio-cognitive abilities (see sidebar on p. 16 for more on zooanthropology).

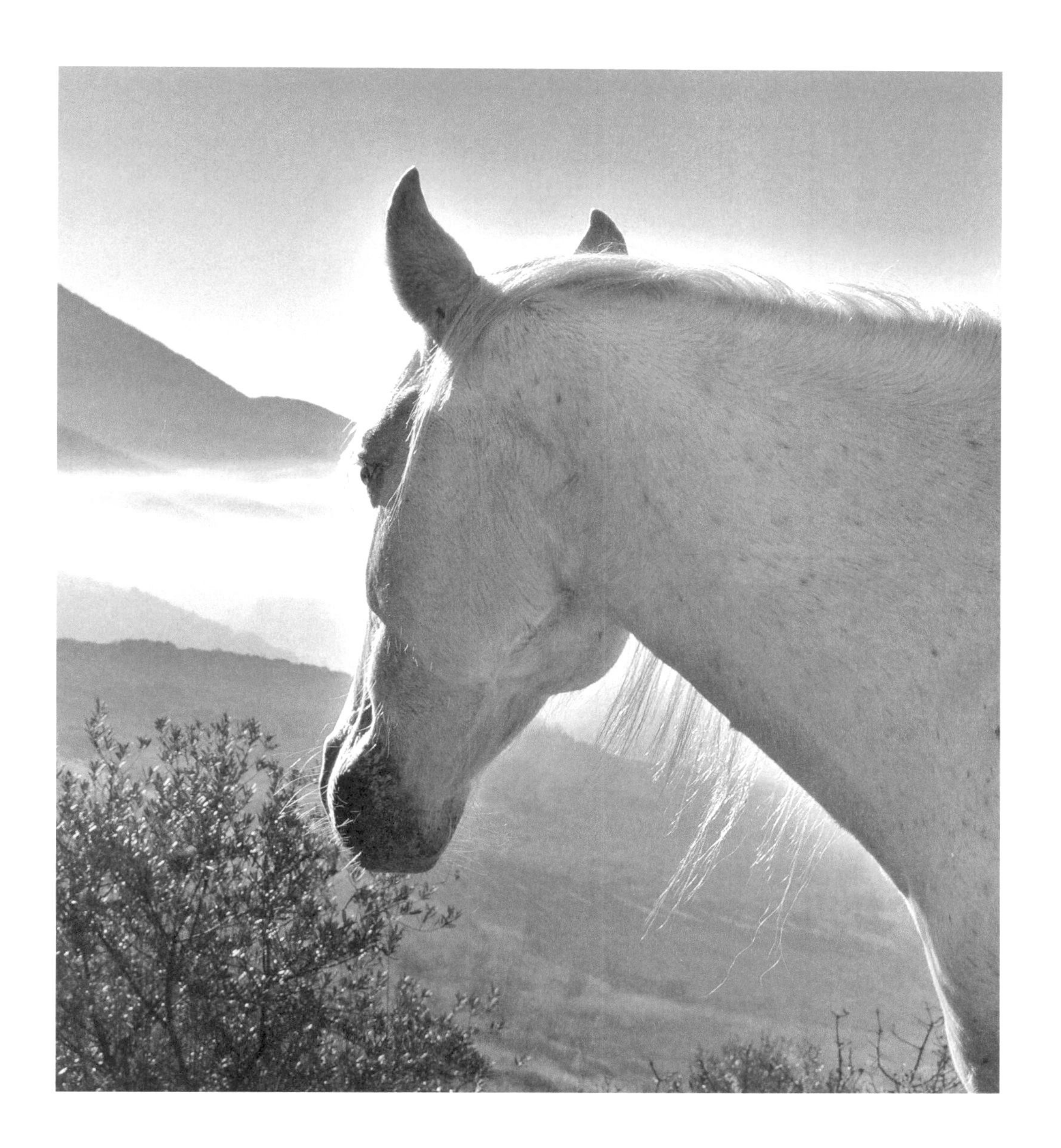

It isn't an easy journey because it chips away many of the universal beliefs we hold in our relationships with horses and other animals. It makes us question ourselves, our automatic and routine behavior when dealing with horses, but also our relationships in general. At the same time, it creates room for greater expression, inspiration, and new insight.

▶ *Understanding animals and human interaction with animals is often seen from an anthropocentric view.*

Indeed, it could be of great benefit to students who want to learn about cognition, emotions, and social-learning aspects; teachers who want to offer their students a different point of view; horse lovers who would like to know more about interspecies-relationships; horse owners wanting to understand socio-cognitive herd dynamics; people interested in a different message; professionals curious about the importance of cognitive ability and affiliated behavior; equine scientists who want to go a step further in the research of equine quality of life; and people interested in the development of human coexistence with other animals.

The journey to understanding the cognitive horse has already astonished people, brought greater awareness and improved their lives as well as their horses. It has made many people "come home," and their horses along with them. It has enabled them to see the "Other" horse—not the one that they have created with their expectations and anthropocentric (considering human beings as the most significant entity of the universe) projections, but the one that has been there all the time, waiting for them to shed their ideas of dominance and hierarchy and their desire for control, which is only an illusion anyway. Indeed, it is only then that people can learn again how to give room to free expression and be able to get to know the horse for what he really is, and always has been.

This book is divided into three parts; each addresses the cognitive horse from a different angle. Part I, "The Invisible Horse," explains how our human beliefs and assumptions have an impact on our perception and how that plays a part in making the horse "invisible" as a cognitive animal. It also shows how the large number of elements that support

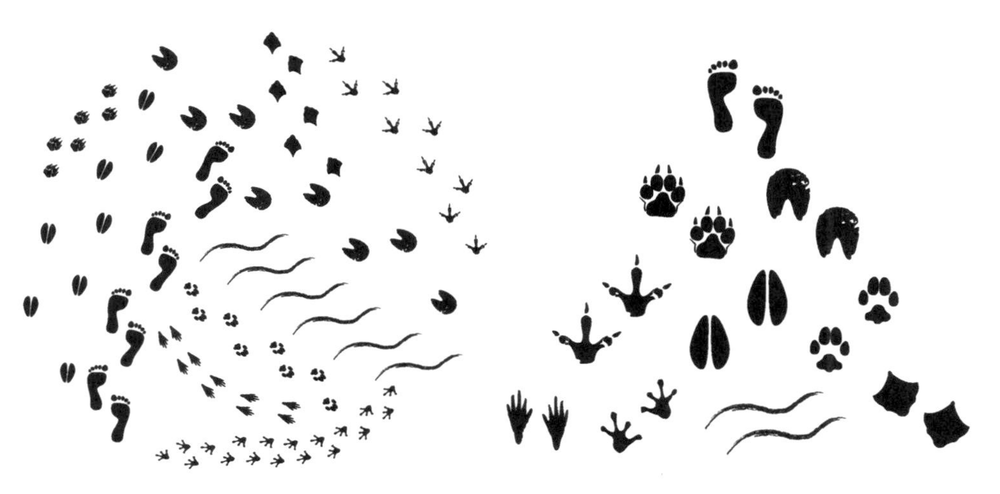

The Zooanthropological Approach *The Anthropocentric Approach*

the current universal idea we have about horses makes it more difficult to allow for observation of relationship dynamics from a different perspective.

Part II, "A Life without Tension," introduces the concepts of equine zooanthropology. It describes what happens when a horse grows up in a socio-cognitive context and what it means for the interaction between horses and humans when these abilities are taken into account. Practical examples are given of horses and their owners who find their way "back" together to a reciprocal relationship.

In Part III, "Growing Together," the human elements are described, as well as the awareness that is necessary to be able to understand the dynamics that are involved in the relationship between horse and human where the cognition of both is taken into account. It talks about letting go of the habits and thought-mechanisms that create many expectations in our interaction with animals. It also helps to understand where the control issue starts, and how we can go back from a need for control to the perception of contact. With that, it will explain the benefit of developing an eye for detail, and creating a better awareness of our senses again. Sharing moments and experiences with horses needs room for expression, as does understanding nuances in relationship dynamics and behavior.

Herd dynamics, and every unique equine-human relationship, are not defined with hierarchic protocol, but depend on the surroundings, inner motivation, and social context of previous experiences and many other elements. This makes every relationship a lifelong journey of shared experiences and discovery.

Thank you for caring about the cognitive horse.

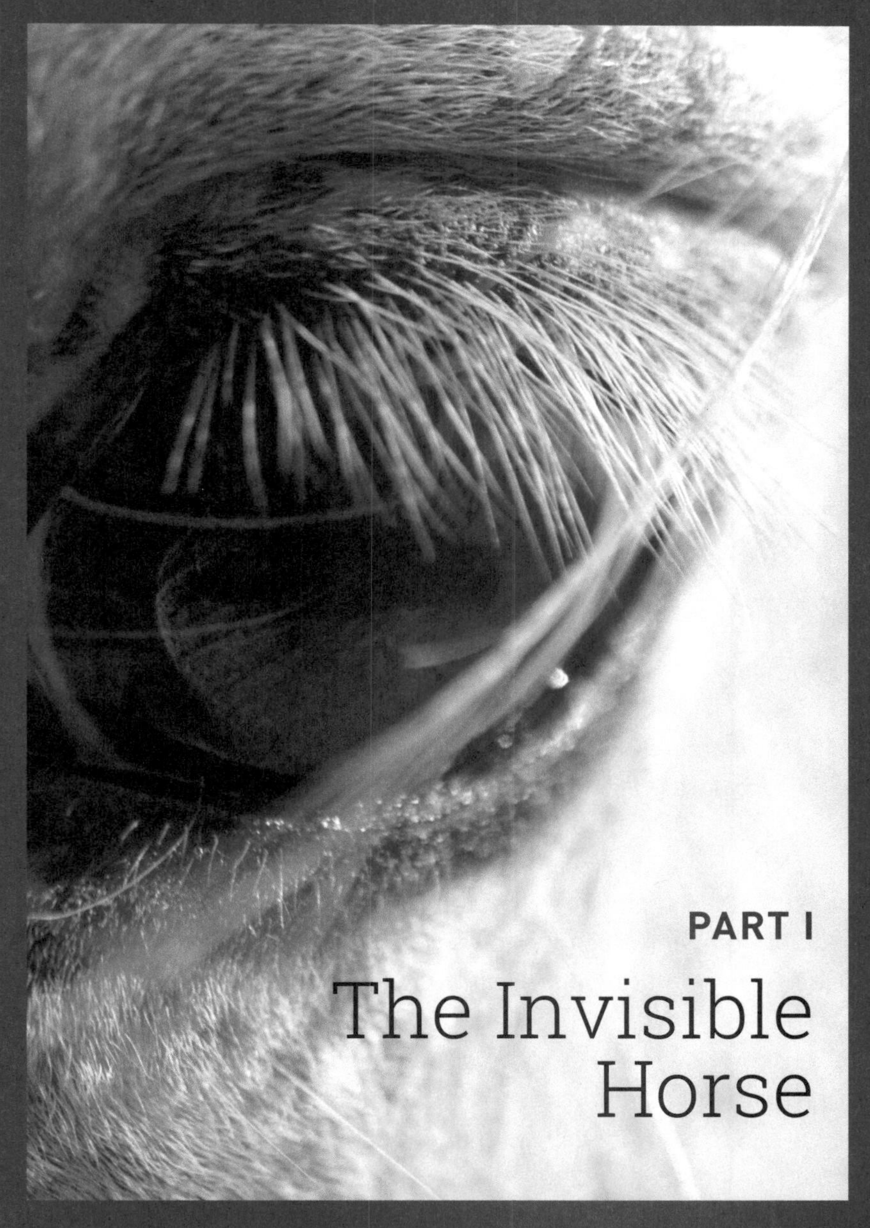

PART I
The Invisible Horse

"The real voyage of discovery consists—not in seeking new landscapes—but in having new eyes. See the universe through the eyes of another, of a hundred others, to see the hundred universes that each of them sees, that each of them is." —Marcel Proust

1

What Is Cognition?

Looking for the Horse

> *It is early in the morning at the end of the summer. On the steep hills of Monte Cairo in Southern Lazio in Italy where the forest thins out to make way for the more barren higher altitude vegetation, the temperature is already rising. It is going to be another hot day.*

We wrote these observations during a summer visit to the Esperia Ponies that live in this region of Italy on the vast plateaus. They have lived here for centuries. They survive in a harsh equilibrium, having to share their natural habitat with wolves whose call one can often hear, and face extreme weather conditions. In the winter, when several feet of snow can fall, they move down to lower ground to seek shelter and forage in a different environment. Similarly, in the summer, at the hottest time of the day, when high temperatures reach even the higher mountain peaks, the horses need to move away from the higher grounds to find shade. Although they get part of their daily water supply from the morning dew, every other day they also need to look for water pools farther down the hills when the higher reserves have run out.

There is a steep meandering path going up between the rocks and trees, and their barefoot hoof prints are clearly visible on the karstic ground—an irregular limestone region. These are traces of the Esperia. This type of ground is one of the reasons why it is hard to find water here at this time of year, because every single raindrop that falls on it sinks into the ground before being distributed through underground sinkholes and streams to hidden caves.

Animals that live in this territory have to take this drought into account to be able to make decisions about when and where to look for water. Their problem-solving capacity needs to be fully operative.

As we sit in a small clearing not far from the edge of the forest, we hear a sudden clattering of steps on stones coming from somewhere behind the higher line of trees. Then, much closer, there is a movement of branches and two horses appear. Two adult mares, strong and robust, with their typical dark coats, come forward. They stop to look at the two of us, sitting motionless, a short distance from the small track. Behind them, standing still among the trees, are other horses. They must be on their way to a water hole somewhere down the path. A couple of minutes go by. They move a little farther forward, followed by the rest of the family, then stop once again to continue observing. There is no snorting or head movements, no tension in their bodies. There is only a pondered observation of the human presence—an unknown element in a known territory.

It is a decision-making process to choose whether to continue along this path to the water or not. Minutes seem to last forever as nothing obvious seems to happen. Then they decide to slowly turn around and the family members behind them turn around as well, one by one, as the intention is passed on, and they disappear once again behind the trees.

But then, from the side of the group, other movements take place.

A very old mare appears. She is clearly weak and has difficulty walking, but is heading steadily in the opposite direction again to the rest of the herd. She passes us. Although her body is old and consumed by the experiences of a lifetime, her gaze is vivid and serene, and that is how she looks at us. Aware of our presence, but not influenced by it, she continues down the path at her strenuous yet steady pace. The other horses remain indecisive for a moment—they look at her, they look at us, they look back up. Then they turn around again as well, all together, and follow the small track down the hill toward the water.

Pleasure Before Pleasure

Spring in the Netherlands, a hot dry wind on April 20, 2014. I leave the house to go outside and to observe the horses in the paddock, taking time to understand their internal state.

With me I have a brush and a currycomb. These are days of massage and grooming to help the horses lose their winter coat. They observe each other, comfortably close to one another in the knowledge that they will all be part of this grooming moment. I also have a saddle, saddle blanket, and halter with me. While massaging and scratching Falò, with the other males around us, I put the saddle blanket on Sparta, the saddle on Fulmine, and the halter on the back of Topazio. We are all merged, blended, and assimilated in the same experience.

Sparta then pulls the saddle off Fulmine's back and the halter off Topazio. While the saddle simply stays where it was dropped, I collect the halter from the ground and put it on Falò, continuing to massage him. Then I pick up the saddle and put it gently on Sparta's back, while scratching his neck and he expresses enjoyment with his head a bit raised and his upper lip moving. Next I take everything off Sparta, putting the blanket on Falò, the saddle on the ground, while Topazio approaches us, backing toward me to be scratched near his tail. I scratch him, then take the saddle from the

Some of the more curious horses look at us, others do not. Having changed their idea of looking for an alternative track, they now proceed along the original path, pass us, and together, move on, listening to the inner motivation of the old and frail mare.

Esperia Ponies have played an important role in the further understanding of equine behavior and horses' rich social dimensions and cognitive abilities. Indeed, their habitat, origins, as well as their daily experiences with each other and their environment, have enabled them

ground and gently put it on the back of Falò, securing it, but loosely. I move away to continue grooming Sparta, who is exploring the saddle's horn, nibbling it, while Falò is almost asleep.

I then groom and massage Fulmine and Topazio, while Falò starts moving around us, all in the same open space, all calm, relaxed, and carefree, all interested in the pleasure and the experience. I tighten the saddle's cinch and mount Falò to simply sit on his back, enjoying the wind that stirs my hair and the horses' tails and manes, continuing to scratch Falò's back, comb his mane with my hand, and massage the other horses, who, in turn, move around me and Falò.

The group movements gradually bring us near the gate of the horses' pasture. I get off Falò, undo the cinch and take off the saddle by sliding it from his back and resting it on the back of Fulmine. I put the blanket on Sparta, and while taking of the halter I turn to lay it on Topazio's back.

Next, I gently slide everything from their backs and put the items on the ground, where they all start exploring the material, incorporated with traces of the pleasant experience, with an internal state of calm. I explore along with them and after a few minutes I open the gate and they all go out in the same relaxed way for some grazing.

I do simple things like that.

to preserve their cognitive essence. They do not react to something without thinking about the situation first. These horses played a central role in the first studies of understanding mental maps and spatial reasoning ability in equids, and they also encouraged further studies about the animal-human interaction. Indeed, their problem-solving capabilities, and their calm decision-making boosted the desire to understand and unravel this "Other" horse as described earlier in this book, making the cognitive horse visible again as a balanced sentient being, instead of merely a reactive horse labelled by the "fight-or-flight" paradigm.

From an evolutionary point of view, horses are mammals and belong to the equid family of the *Perissodactyla* order (hooved mammals). From an ecological point of view, horses are herbivores and can be subject to predation by certain carnivore species, depending where they live. From an ethological (study of animal behavior under natural conditions) point of view, horses are socio-cognitive animals in their specific and individual patterns. Thinking of them merely in terms of prey or "fight-or-flight" animals is clearly too simple and doesn't make it possible for us to see them as they truly are.

Many modern training methods, however, focus on this simplistic concept that horses are flight and reactive animals that need to be controlled if we want a safe and efficient interaction. In reality, they become fight-or-flight animals as a result of their coexistence with humans. In the story of the encounter with the Esperia Ponies, for example, there is no sign of a flight tendency. There is no need for it. So what we should ask ourselves is why domestic horses feel the need to show so many reactive behaviors.

All horses are born cognitive. Their cognitive abilities allow them to understand themselves, their initiatives, each other, their environment, and their social context. However, due to their coexistence with humans, horses gradually change because not only do they usually grow up in a context in which the elements that make a socio-cognitive environment have vanished, but they also start to fulfill a human purpose. They start to respond to stimuli with behavioristic responses without actually processing the information. It is not surprising that what we then see is an unpredictable flight animal.

Perceiving horses as flight animals is a deep-rooted belief that influences many aspects of human behavior toward them. It is present in a wide range of situations. Here is a simple example: Someone leads a horse out to a field. At the moment the halter is taken off—or the rope is detached from the halter—the horse gallops away. If the horse doesn't run away, he is often given a "friendly" tap on his rump or an arm is waved to encourage him to charge off. But why should he run? And if he doesn't run off, why do so many of us feel the need to trigger that reaction? As a symbol for freedom, perhaps? This is just one of the many moments in which horses, in their coexistence with us, are pushed into adopting a reactive behavior.

Due to these habits and beliefs, many of the ideas in the horse world (whether scientific ones or folk knowledge) are based on the calibration of a behavior pattern that is formed and influenced by a context that man has created for horses, and the experiences he has forced them to live. The fact that we can then see their reactive responses just reinforces the assumption that horses need strict and clear rules to avoid confusion—that they need humans to take charge.

The point is that horses become helpless and reactive animals in an interaction that does not take into account the horse. If we want to meet their needs, develop their true inner potential, and allow for quality of life, we need to change our approach. Instead of the current focus on their physical potential and understanding how to exploit them (we try to make them run faster, jump higher, lift their knees higher, trot extremely long distances, and more, all in line with the distorted view man has of them), we need to create opportunities for them to experience and understand their own life—even the most minute details of their living habitat—and create room for an inter-species dialogue.

2

Cognition Comes Naturally

What Is Cognition?

So what do we mean by cognition in horses? What do we mean by cognition in general?

Cognition is a faculty that processes information, applies knowledge, and changes preferences. It is both how the world is perceived and the knowledge that is derived from that perception (i.e. mental representations of the world). Attention, memory, problem-solving, and decision-making are all key elements within the cognitive processes.

Trying to understand and explain the mental abilities of animals (human animals included) often creates discussion because there are several very different definitions of cognition that relate to how people, including scientists, look at the world. The *anthropocentric* view, for instance, places human intelligence and cognition at the top of a pyramid, and tends to compare the abilities of other animals with human ones. The field of study called *zooanthropology,* on the other hand, stresses the value of different forms of cognition.

Here is an example to illustrate these differences and their consequences: The use of language and the solving of mathematical problems are easily recognizable cognitive processes in humans. It is, therefore, tempting to apply the same processes to horses: teach them how to count, recognize numbers or the alphabet, then use the results as evidence of a form of equine intelligence. However, a horse that is able to count has actually learned a trick. It gives a misleading picture of the true capacity and needs of the horse and belittles his essence, especially when it is achieved with food premiums, as these take away the focus from the horse's actual understanding of a context.

Learning the human alphabet is not of interest to a horse. It is, however, gratifying to man to train a horse to perform such a task. What is interesting to a horse is being able to understand his surroundings, spatial representations, social dynamics, problem-solving situations, or pre-conflict (where one horse interrupts two others that are starting a conflict) and consolatory (consoling) behaviors.

A horse doesn't need a reward for this, because as an inner need and motivation, being given a premium for explorative behavior would be an antithesis. His satisfaction is an intrinsic one that is derived from the possibility to elaborate (work out carefully or minutely) information.

Trying to prove intelligence by creating behavioral projections from the human world, or trying to compare capacities instead of understanding different cognitive abilities, creates confusion in the awareness of what animal cognition really means. It also creates filters in our ability to see the intrinsic value of a particular animal, of an individual.

Equine Cognition

In nature, a horse is a cognitive animal because life in the wild preserves cognitive abilities. Equine cognition has also been shaped by the evolutionary process, both by the environmental challenges and horses' complex social dynamics. In fact, every species, and every individual within that species, has his own particular cognitive abilities and skills. Bats and spiders, for example, have a particularly developed spatial cognition that allows them to navigate through and hunt in their environment.

In *Animal Cognition in Nature* (Academic Press, 1998), Russell P. Balda, Irene M. Peppenberg, and Alan C. Kamil say: "We have long since left the realm where animals are viewed as simple, stimulus-bound responders, passive learners or robotic followers of conditioning regimes."

Sadly, in today's society, this concept doesn't seem to be recognized yet for the equine species. Think for example of the situation when a horse is taken to a new habitat. Many horses are expected to immediately adapt without giving them the opportunity or creating possibilities for them to explore and get to know this new environment. Although the new place is full

▶ *Just because we are not looking, or not asking him to do something, doesn't mean a horse stops perceiving his world.*

Zooanthropology

The study field of zooanthropology includes several scientific, philosophical, and political disciplines. Zooanthropology defines and gives direction within the interpretation of phenomena related to our relationship with other animals, stepping outside the anthropocentric viewpoint. It is not just a matter of study and application; it gives an ethical direction and inspires a movement for years to come. It refers to the cognitive ethology dimension, and does not fall into the dimension of classical ethology or behaviorism.

Zooanthropology recognizes the nonhuman "Other" as a subject and, for this, clearly disapproves of the use of coercive instruments, whether physical, emotional, or mental, and certainly calls into question all tools, methods, and approaches regarding the interpretation and application of operant conditioning. It questions animal training, and opens up a new model of interpretation and application in the dynamics of animal learning, recognizing animal subjectivity and alterity ("Otherness").

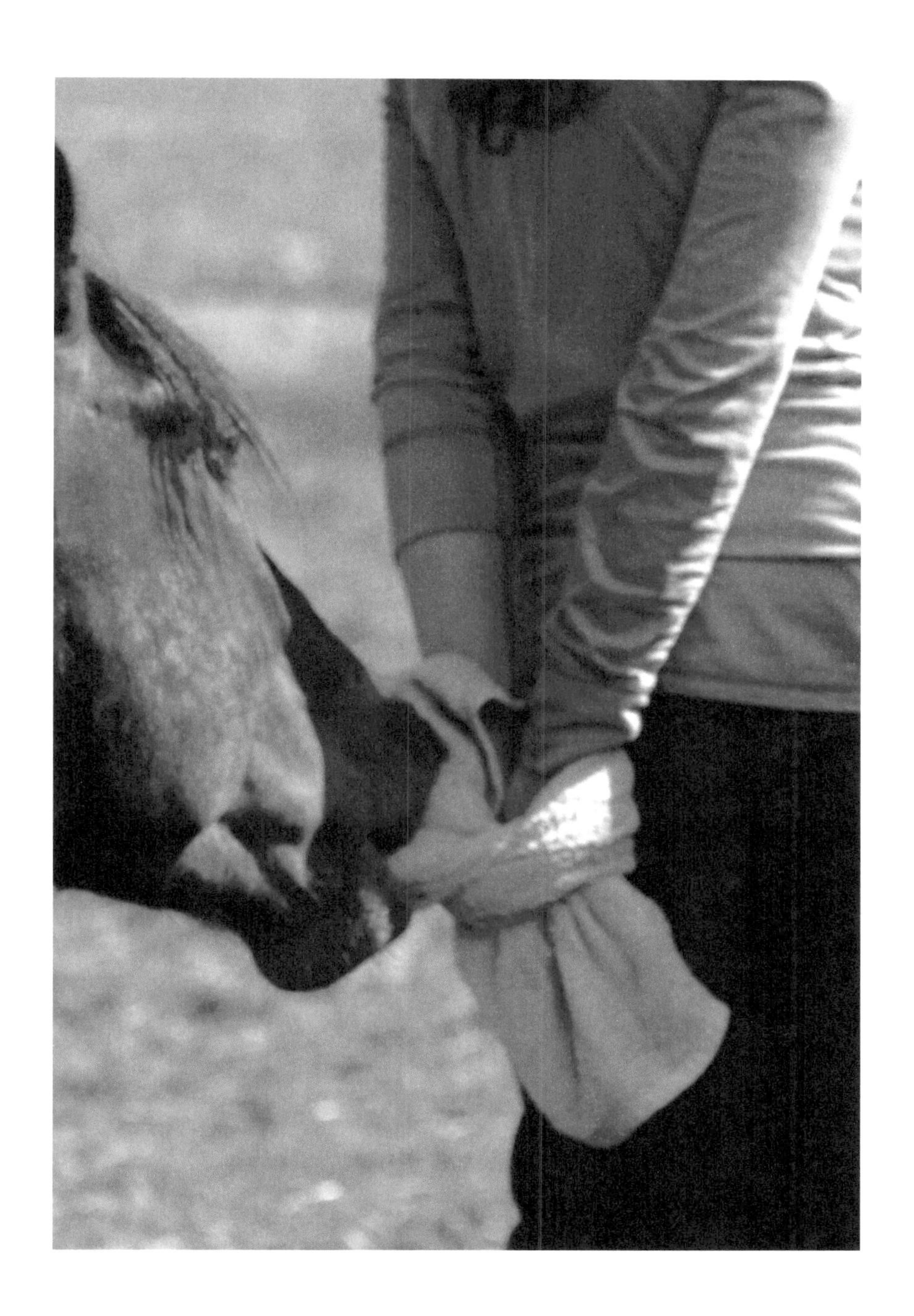

of information for the horse, we do not perceive these elements as learning opportunities. As a result, many horses live in a blurred world full of situations and interactions they just get used to seeing but don't really understand. Even the saddle is a completely unknown object for most horses.

Besides recognizing and accepting their need to explore—for example, a new environment—we also need to recognize the information acquisition process as something that belongs to the horse. Thus, we might not see any result or get any evidence of what the learning has brought because one of the characteristics of cognitive learning is latency, which means that often we cannot see the immediate result of the learning process; what was elaborated might be used in a future moment, if and when necessary, as when circumstances call for it. However, even if we do not see the result of the elaboration process, what we can do is create room for learning.

▶ *Exploring in a cognitive context is a calm and calming process.*

This is a problem for other animals, as well. Think of a cat going outside for the first time. Most cats will sit on the doorstep first, at the limit between their secure environment and the unknown, taking time to observe everything and form an idea of the situation. The human companion, however, is often too impatient because he wants to see some action and a result. So he interrupts that process and tries to convince the cat to step out. We need to learn to recognize and respect these learning moments instead.

Cognition and Well-Being

Although the understanding of animal cognition has become an important topic and a crucial element for the horse's quality of life, still relatively little is known about it.

We must, therefore, let go of the Cartesian and performative approach in a scientific context as it is too reductionist and often at the service of the equestrian world: this approach is focused on how to

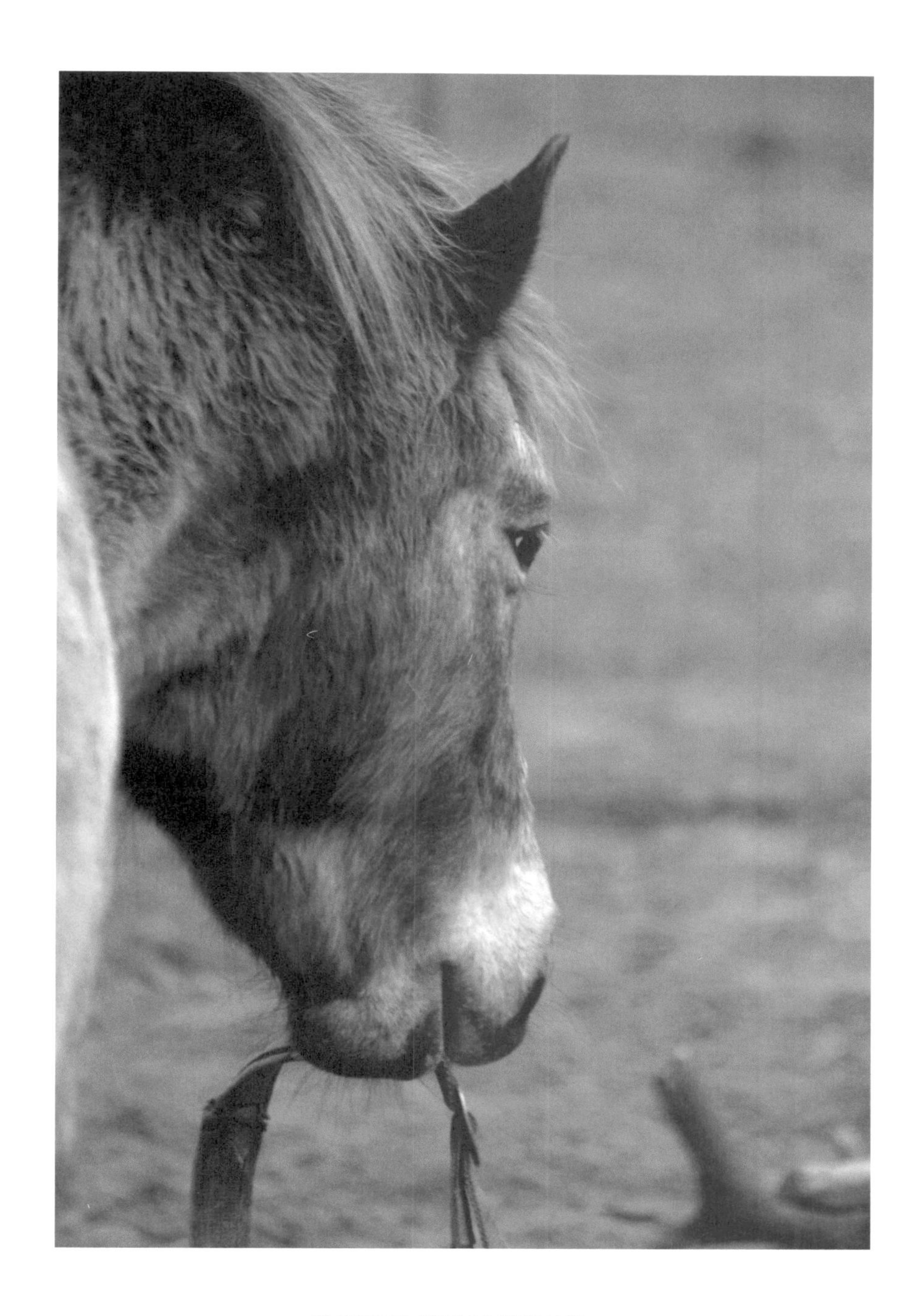

Getting to Know Each Other

Equine dynamics, in a balanced socio-cognitive context, are mostly moments of calm understanding. The fact that we see fights whenever horses are first put together tells more about how their social abilities have been impacted by humans and how the process of integration is not preserving their actual needs.

Yesterday, the neighbor's horses' paddock was changed. The Friesian foal, his mother, and the Shetland mare found themselves alongside our mare group, with whom they have been neighbors for a while. On the other side were our four males—the bachelor band. For the males, this was a moment of strong interest. The four of them stood next to each other, observing and taking everything in. For the females, this was a new situation where they could exchange information. In a balanced socio-cognitive context it is not about hierarchy and dominance, understanding who has which rank. They are not an army.

▶ *Every horse should have the possibility, driven by his own inner curiosity, to smell, touch, explore, taste, and feel whatever is part of his surroundings.*

Getting to know each other is about understanding, elaborating information, taking it one step at the time to be able to take each other into account. Creating an image of each other, and of the relationship dynamics as well, starts beyond a fence.

This means, for example, that in one moment, the Shetland mare showed a bit of an exaggerated, reactive behavior toward the foal (with a rear kick), while our male Falò actually expressed a soft, calming nickering.

The usual interpretation would have been that the Shetland mare claimed dominance toward the foal. But the Shetland mare in that situation is actually in need of a more slow understanding of the dynamics around her, of new experiences in which she finds she can actually trust and rely upon the horses around her being able to read dynamics and herself.

A balanced herd searches for a calm life together and preserves each member's inner state.

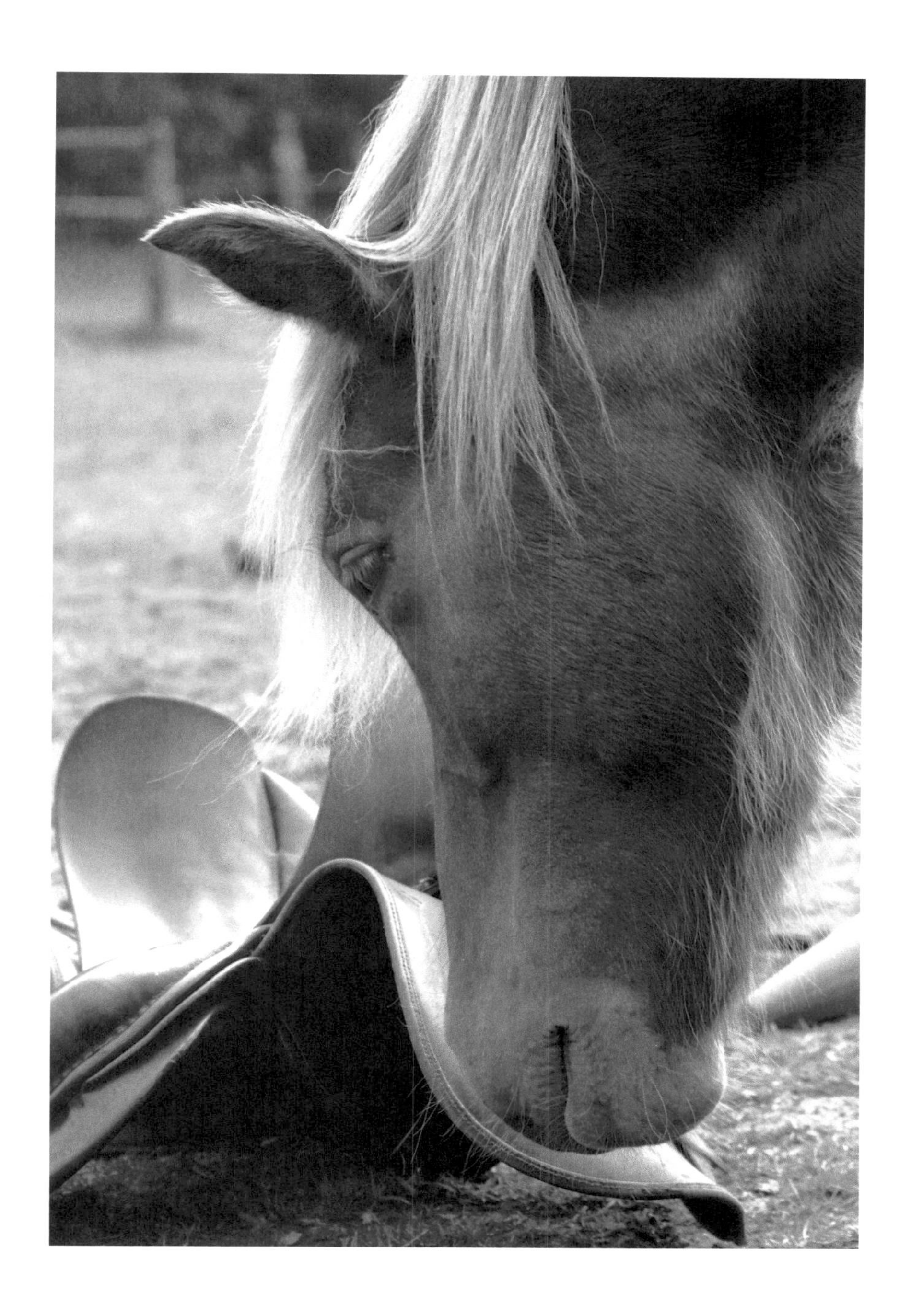

train a horse, rather than how to understand his needs and preserve his socio-cognitive abilities.

Welfare, well-being, and cognition are closely linked. Ignoring cognition means ignoring a horse's profound and innate need to understand what is happening around him, understand his environment, and elaborate and express his own experience. Ignoring it will cause tension in the horse, mentally, emotionally, and physically. Yet, the more we study horse cognition from a human point of view, the less we know about his real emotional, social, and mental perception and understanding. We need to study horse cognition in a new way.

▶ *Every relationship is unique.*

What Is a Cognitive Environment?

Horses that live in a social context and an enriched natural environment live in the context of social experience and learning. Their social dynamics, observation, and processing of information are continuous: they perform them while foraging, walking together, standing still together, and looking at what another horse is noticing, for example.

As in other species, horses living in a family context have their own cultural transmission. The fact of knowing each other, experiencing moments together, and having the freedom to express themselves, gives horses from a family, or family-like group, a detailed reading of each other that enables them to pick up on each other's intentions by watching each other and doing things together. Refined social interactions such as pre-conflict behavior, affiliative behavior (behavior that promotes group cohesion), and shared exploring are then also developed. They take social dynamics into account and, in doing so, safeguard a cognitive context.

Horses can share experiences, and learn together and from each other. A young horse can learn by observing a mature, experienced horse, but a mature horse can also learn from a young horse.

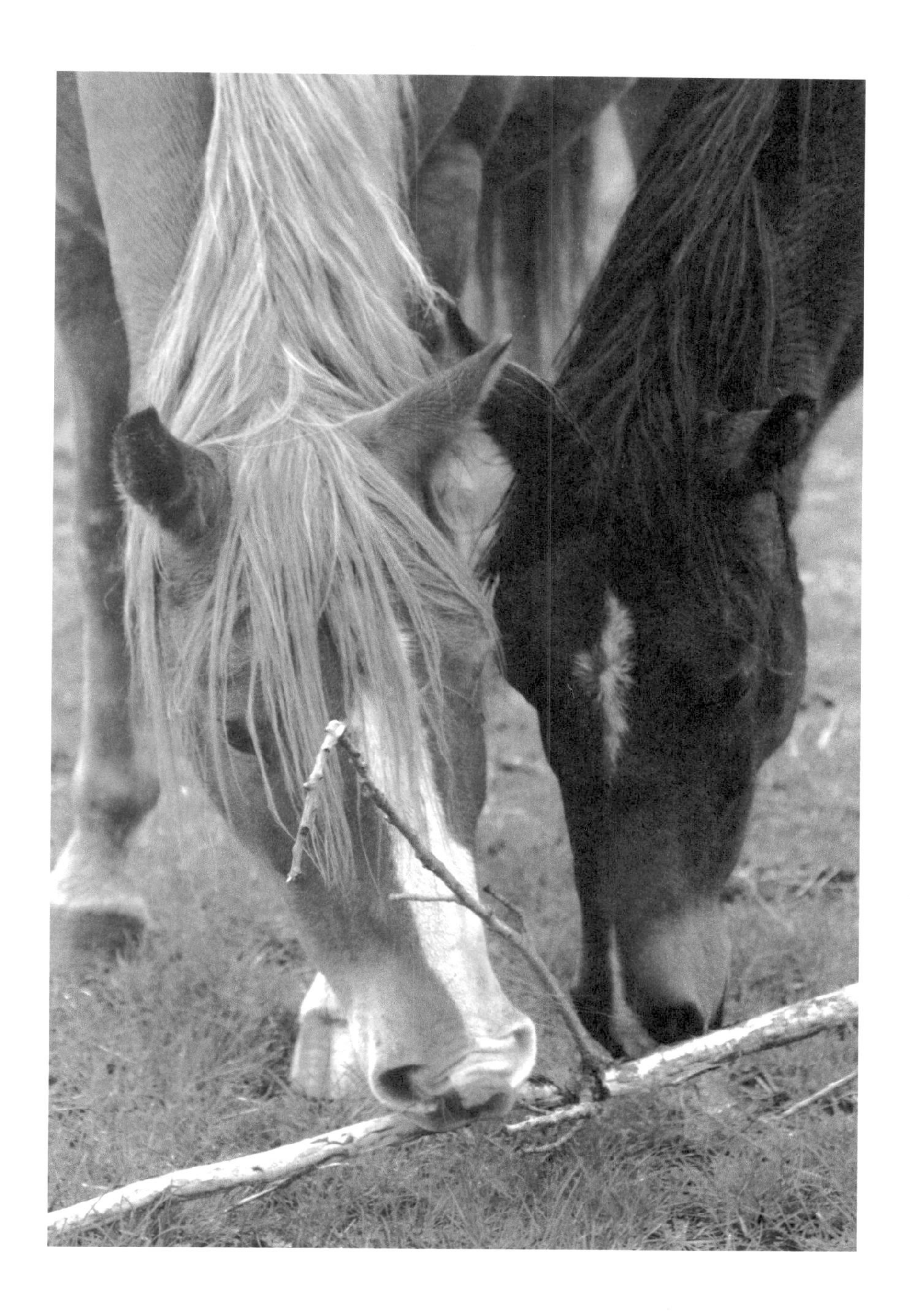

It is called social learning in a socio-cognitive context. In this context, living together means living experiences together, learning nuanced expressions in a kind of dialogue in which every single relationship is unique and in continuous development. Obviously, the richness of these experiences depends on the individual horses involved. Similarly, if the environment becomes too dynamic, too competitive, or if there are no elements that support the shared experiencing, the conditions for socio-cognitive learning decrease.

Having shared experiences is crucial in creating a cognitive environment that gives the possibility for a deeper understanding of the context and of each other, not only for a young horse, but for every horse, for every relationship. However, it is also important to understand that putting a number of horses together doesn't automatically mean that a safe social environment is created. Most horses in our society have no family ties or family-like groups in their living habitat and do not grow up together.

Preserving Socio-Cognitive Abilities

Living together in the same field is not the same as having shared experiences in a socio-cognitive context, especially when there are continuous changes. In many situations, horses are busy defending themselves, rather than trying to understand each other.

Humans can play an important role by creating the opportunities for horses to share social experiences with each other, such as facilitating an exploration in the field. Horses are often exposed instead to fast dynamics: many owners go into a field to directly take a horse out, not to spend time in the field and notice from nearby what kind of environment and dynamics their horse-companion is living in.

Cognition can only be preserved in a context where there is respect for the specific ethological needs. However, this is not sufficient. Preserving cognition and cognitive structures also means avoiding elements that could cause reactive experiences, such as:

- Premature weaning of the foal
- Social isolation
- Living in a non-familiar group or experiencing frequent changes (even with known horses)
- Living under pressure or with performance expectations
- Behavioristic training
- The use of bits, spurs, shoeing
- No room for explorative moments in interactions with man
- Result-driven human monologue with no room for equine self-expression

Preserving cognitive abilities means ensuring a cognitive context in which a horse will live. It is a context where there is respect for the horse's specific ethological needs, but also where he can express himself, understand his environment, and where he isn't continuously exposed to pressure and expectations in his interactions with humans. However, nowadays, most horses experience stressful situations from the moment they are born. The premature weaning of foals, social isolation, life in non-familiar and unstable groups, behavioristic training, and a performance-oriented human lifestyle all strongly impact their cognitive structures and their welfare.

As social cognition is strongly related to the perception of each individual horse, and depends on all the previously mentioned elements, we need to learn to see a horse in this complex situation. We need to adopt a more holistic approach in understanding a relationship dynamic that cannot be captured by or attained with a method. That would be like finding a method for a happy human-human relationship. Although many may have actually tried to capture it in a formula, in the end, we still have to experience every single relationship. And that is the beauty of it! Every sound relationship is a unique interaction in continuous evolution. With every new experience, everyone grows and acquires new instruments with which to see and perceive life.

A relationship that lasts and is based on cognition cannot be put in a manual as if it were a machine or a mathematical equation. It requires an awareness of all the various elements within the relationship dynamic.

3
Self-Fulfilling Prophecies

Why Do Horses Spook?

The view (and misunderstanding) that the horse is a reactive animal is kept alive by the fact that nearly everything linked to the horse is based on the idea previously explained—that "he is a fight-or-flight animal." It is the first phrase that makes everything else difficult to unravel. Books, blogs, videos, training DVDs—the message is constant and insistent: "Why does a horse spook? He spooks because it is the most natural thing for him to do."

But it is not.

It is what humans think is the most natural thing for him to do. When a horse spooks, instead of asking, "Where did I go too far?" or, "What can I do differently?" the question usually asked is, "How can I make him stop spooking?" We start to desensitize and expose the horse, with pressure and food rewards, to other strange objects, hoping to train him until he no longer shows any flight reaction. Yet the problem remains. That horse has not actually been able to understand the context, and will spook again as circumstances change. And, once again, we will not be surprised by his behavior because we think it's just the way horses are. However, a horse isn't only evaluating everything from a black-and-white perspective, needing to decide whether something is dangerous or not. A horse can also just be intrigued, for the simple fact that gathering information is interesting. The outcome might not lead to a reaction, but the information is stored as knowledge, processed somewhere to help in making a decision, or simply kept for future applications—or not.

Here is an example to show how easily we can ignore a horse's need for understanding: Consider a young Fjord named Tommy, already fully trained to the saddle and ridden despite his young age of three. This is what his owner says of him: "It is wonderful to ride out with Tommy. He is so brave. He learned so fast. It's too bad that he made a habit of spooking near the other paddocks every time we leave the stable."

▶ *A social context should facilitate every new experience, as no horse-human interaction should be based on taking a horse out of his comfort zone.*

Until the age of two, Tommy had been a balanced, curious, and explorative horse. He lived in a pasture with another young colt. He used to look around, observe the other horses in their paddocks, learn about the different soils, the water, and discover all the other elements in his surroundings.

Then he was trained for riding, taken out of his habitat without allowing him to make this new experience truly his own. It was done without taking his rhythms or his physical and emotional growth into consideration. It ignored his need for a social environment with other horses, as well as the possibility of sharing an experience and exploring new things. As a result, Tommy now has difficulty understanding his surroundings. He is not sure what he is going to do or what he will be asked to do. The paddocks and other elements of his surroundings, which were first a safe haven, have now become a reason to spook. A habit? No. It is just a constant reminder for Tommy that he doesn't feel secure.

So does a horse with preserved and developed cognitive abilities

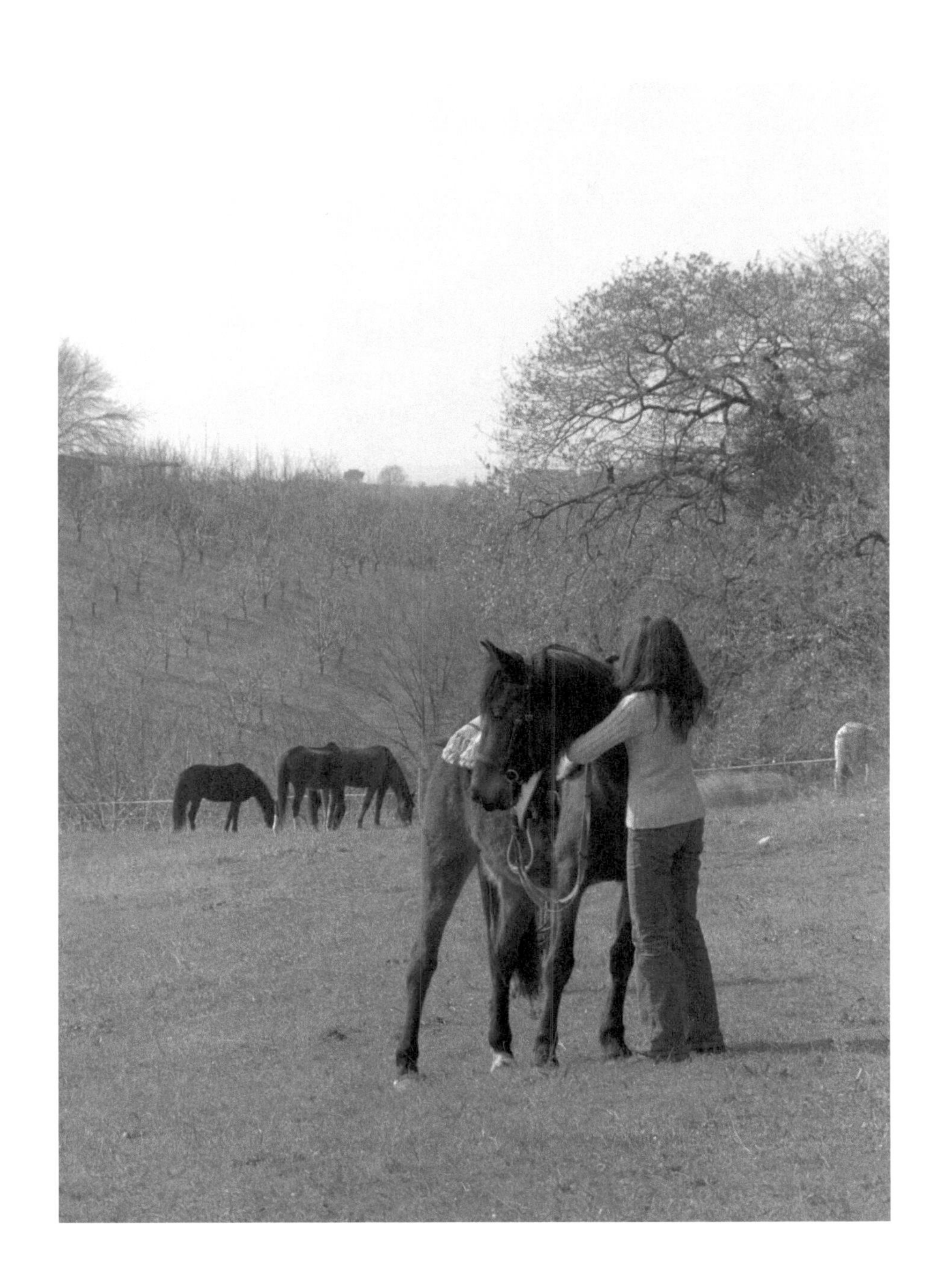

ever get scared and jump up when something really strange happens?

If you see something strange and unexpected as a human, you might be alarmed, and so might a horse. As an example, think of a piece of a flapping canvas placed over some wood near a paddock. This situation would generate curiosity in a cognitive horse; he would look at it, integrate it into his mental map, and then proceed. A reactive horse, on the other hand, would jump away and remain in a state of tension and suspicion for several more minutes, even from a distance. The cognitive horse follows the same rule as all living beings: *Minimal effort, maximum result.*

▶ *You can bring a horse to "your environment" or bring "your environment" to the horse.*

To improve equine well-being, it is extremely important to understand a horse's cognitive needs, learn how we can develop and enhance our coexistence with him, and how we can share activities in ways that don't make him reactive.

There is still a lot of focus on the horse's *physical* welfare. Despite the fact that, in research, there is growing awareness that horses have social-learning skills and higher mental abilities, horse *learning* is still referred to as a simplistic stimulus-response model, with all the practical impacts this has on man's perception of the horse.

The Machine-Animal

Thinking about and trying to define what non-human animals are and what differentiates their minds from human-animal minds are questions that go far back in history. Aristotle defined the human being as "the rational animal," and by doing so, established rationality as the distinguishing factor between man and all other animals. Centuries later, Descartes defined animals as "soulless machines." According to him, animal behavior could be explained without the existence of a thought process or consciousness. He also ignored the possibility of differences between individuals in non-human animals. Then, at the end of the eighteenth century, Kant stated that animals only have an

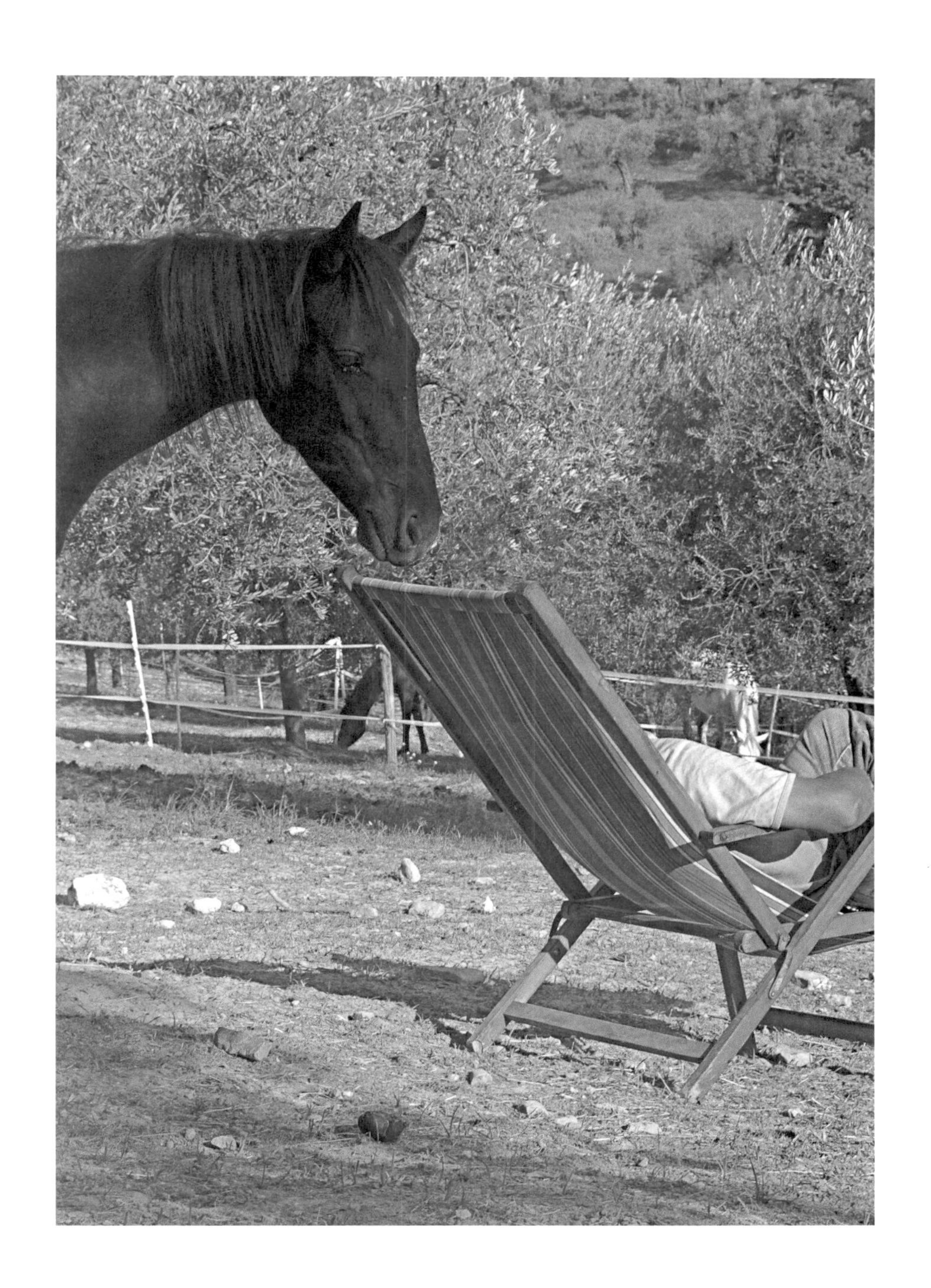

instrumental value and cannot think for themselves because they are not rational beings.

Today, the ideas put forward by these philosophical debates still linger in many animal-related studies and activities, making it all the more difficult to study animal cognition with an open mind. The perception of an object-machine-animal also perpetuates the tendency to interpret behavior as a response to a stimulus, which explains why behaviorism is still the most common approach when analyzing animal behavior.

However, instead of a reaction to something, behavior should be interpreted and understood as the way an experience is lived and perceived. Horses need information and comprehension to be able to connect with themselves and the world around them (including other horses and humans). We need to stop representing the horse's mind as a black box that is unable to create its own representation of a certain situation. It is not a machine that only gives an output (behavior) when a certain order is given. The consequences of ignoring the cognitive and emotional needs of any sentient being can have a huge impact on his quality of life.

4

Time for a Change

Back in Time

If we want to go back to a time before horses were used by humans, we must go to a period before the first known domestication of the horse, to a prehistoric place where our ancestors first met the equine species and our reciprocal coevolution began. Some of the information they exchanged must have been similar: information they acquired from their senses, their scents, from the weather, from the ground, from their inner states, from group dynamics, from their understanding of reciprocal intents.

Our ancestors painted these animals that shared their environment on the walls of their caves. By doing so, not only did they reproduce in the caves reflections of their natural environment, but they acquired information from these images, thus helping them to understand their own being—also from a socio-cognitive point of view.

The famous horses painted in the Chauvet Cave in France that have been dated from 32,000 to 35,000 years ago seem to be very different from the images we see everywhere today. From this ancient impression, we can imagine an affiliative dimension, where the panel of four horses are emphatically synchronized and clearly represent a social group. Nowadays, however, in sculptures, paintings, and shows, we see a tense horse, in social isolation, which clearly reflects how we have lost the ability recognize his inner state, and even see beauty in the horse's distress. This somehow impacts on our empathic abilities of understanding the "Other."

"The human can only understand himself from the contribution given by the non-human animal."
—Roberto Marchesini

Yet, how did our views of the horse get so entwined with our image of the horse as a tense animal? What happened in his coexistence with humans to generate this altered, reductive, and erroneous image? And what are we doing? Why are we still training and insisting on using past traditions instead of creating room for new understanding and coexistence? Of course, such a change isn't easy. It means understanding the horse's needs, from a well-being point of view, as well as understanding his social dynamics without conditioning his behavior. Most of all, it requires different norms and values for a higher quality of life, where friendship, self-awareness, confidence, expression, and development of his intrinsic value are fundamental key elements.

Changing Awareness

Change is a continuous process. Nothing is immutable. Yet, the universal image we have of horses and the traditional ways we work with them hinder our attempts to create awareness of the horse as a cognitive and sentient being and make this necessary change more difficult to achieve. Indeed, changing is not just recognizing and endorsing other elements, but also letting go of expectations and breaking down schemes and habits. It means understanding how to look at the horse-human relationship from a different perspective.

As an example, let's imagine the situation when we are introducing a foal to the halter. We allow the foal to explore the halter, yet we don't know if his behavior means he is actually accepting it. People often work in terms of "to do's," tasks that need to be achieved. They ask themselves, "Is the foal collaborating, or not? Is he accepting the halter, or not?" Changing our approach in this situation would be to say, "Hey, he's smelling the halter; I wonder what he smells?" We will obviously not get an answer to that question, but we will have become aware of the foal's experience. If we took the time and were curious enough to smell the halter ourselves, we would also get closer to his experience and be able to share the moment with him. But it is very difficult to let go of our own expectations, especially if we are worried the foal might not learn to wear the halter.

The change in perceiving the horse as a cognitive and sentient being is related to various aspects:

- Understanding the horse and being aware of his need for a socio-cognitive environment
- Understanding our difficulty to let go of "to do's" and start working on shared experiences
- Understanding that many horses have been trained in ways that have increased their reactive behavior rather than in ways that give room for shared experiences, allowing for a cognitive state
- Understanding that our expectations and desire for short-term results have a negative impact on the horse-human dialogue that needs, on the contrary, room for expression

It asks for breaking down automatically performed activities and also a change in perception of time. Often both the horse and the human need to learn to break down their routine again (see Part III, p. 85).

The Zooanthropologic Approach

Zooanthropology is a multidisciplinary field of study that analyzes the relationship in which both parties enjoy freedom of expression. This reciprocity is considered a foundation for mutual development and well-being. In the zooanthropologic approach, the human (decentralized as the human) and the non-human animal are a reference for each other (co-learning). Zooanthropology stresses the importance of "Otherness" ("alterity"), the understanding of different cognitive abilities, and the understanding of the "Other" as capable of dialogue and as someone you can learn from.

These elements are brought together in what is called the "affiliative-cognitive paradigm," which takes into account the room for freedom of expression and inner motivation.

Zooanthropology allows us to rediscover the possibility of being in dialogue with the "Otherness," or in this case, with the horse. It enables us to rediscover and develop our awareness in order to use it as a compass in understanding our interactions with others. Zooanthropology offers a different way of looking at animals by taking different aspects into account, but it also implies that we should be curious and must abandon our expectations and our need to control, letting go of the anthropocentric way of looking at human and non-human animal interaction. It is not easy, but at the same time it is also part of our ancient heritage.

"Once the mind has been stretched by a new idea, it will never again return to its original size."
—Oliver Wendell Holmes, Jr.

Equine Zooanthropology

Regarding the horse-human relationship, zooanthropology is not a new horse-training method, but an approach to understanding how a reciprocal relationship can be developed and how we can take the horse's world of perception and his socio-cognitive abilities into account. We need to consider his ability to think, to elaborate, to search for information, to listen to his own motivation, to express emotion or intention, to solve problems, to adapt to changes, and to develop long-lasting relationships. All these elements form the core of any experience, and each one constitutes an experience by itself.

The equine cognitive/zooanthropologic approach is part of a cultural development and evolution that leaves behind the assumption that a horse should be trained and conditioned. In the development of a reciprocal relationship and a socio-cognitive context where horses live and share experiences together, the focus is on the horse's abilities to build latent (not immediately evident) learning experiences himself, which will create a rich living environment for the horse, both in his relationship with other horses and in his relationship with man.

From Object Back to Subject

As many activities that involve human interaction with horses are developed with a focus on the equestrian activities themselves in which the horse is perceived merely as an object, most of the language used adapts to that image. This is logical if we think how closely, in our human perception, the horse is related to a specific activity. Anyone who has a horse, for instance, must have been asked, "What do you do with it?" As a companion animal, a horse is almost always linked to the idea of performing a specific human activity (jumping, dressage, recreational riding, therapeutic riding, as examples). Even in children's books about farm animals, it is not uncommon to see all the other animals as they are (for example, without ear tags), but the horse might still walk around with a halter, a bridle, or sometimes even with a saddle, as if it is intrinsically linked to the horse. We affirm ourselves continuously in an anthropocentric and instrumental perception of horses.

Advertisements state phrases like, "Horses for all circumstances and seasons"; "Training perfect horses for whatever their riders wish"; or "Training a wide variety of horses to become most versatile partners for their new owners." Although probably written by people with a passion for horses, obviously, if this is how we perceive them, the impact on their sentient being is huge. It poses the idea that you would buy a motorbike with an instruction manual, but ignore the individual essence of the horse.

Similarly, if you go to a riding school where children are learning to ride, they might choose the horse of their preferred color. And you can often hear the phrase, "Tell him who's the boss!" The focus is on performance and is done with pressure. When a horse is being ridden and is continuously asked for a response, a strong incentive for reactive behavior is being created. It also creates emotive conflicts in the child and frustration when the animal doesn't respond "correctly." For many children (and adults) the riding school is a strange reality to learn more about horses.

▶ *Being attuned to each other, reading each other's gestures, comes naturally in a reciprocal relationship where intentions are shared. It is not a result of behavioral protocol in a laboratory.*

For what should be taught is *comprehension.* The child should be helped to understand the horse as a social species, with his own interests and fascinating behavior. The problem is that the socio-cognitive abilities of horses are not even taught in the conventional educational system related to horses and horse professionals. So, even if riding schools started teaching about the horse, it would still be based on the necessity to establish control and done from an anthropocentric point of view.

Often explained as necessary for safety reasons,

The Sentient Observer

Close your eyes, so you can open them,
so you can see more clearly.

I do not follow you,
I do not lead you,
I observe you.

I can live that moment of observation,
smell it, grasp it,
elaborate it, learn from it, without
any automatic reactions.

I am a horse, a dog, a cat, a rabbit.
I am a sentient being, are you?

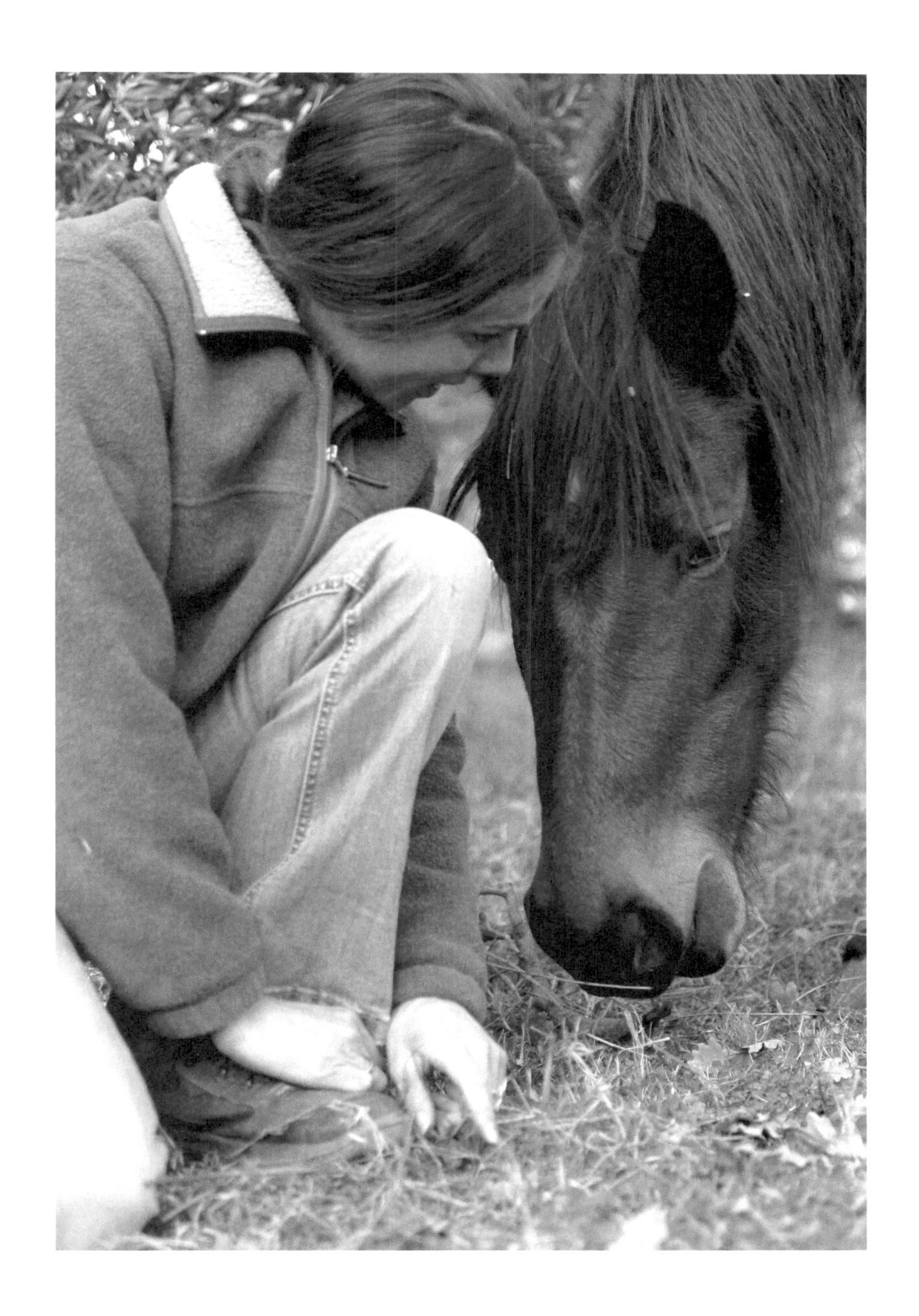

"establishing control" is an important misconception. A horse that is not able to understand who he is or where he is often becomes a time bomb, especially as everything nowadays has to go faster and results need to be reached immediately. We see more and more lost and perplexed expressions on the faces of horses and people going out for a ride.

In a society where the concept of contact is getting more difficult to understand due to our development of technology and communication instruments, children also need to learn about affiliative behavior toward the "Other," whether another human or non-human animal. This cannot be done by asking children to perform a task. Rather, it is done gradually, teaching them first of all how to observe, without expectations or preconceived ideas, and allowing them to experience curiosity toward the "Other." They should be given a context, together with the horse, where both can exchange, where they can develop culture and relationship experiences, where they can listen to their own inner motivation and learn how to listen to others.

▶ *Only when you give horses the space, the context, and the time to create their own experiences, their own learning, their own sharing, and when you focus on their quality of life, will you see the horse as he is.*

Learning how to perceive and how to consider the "Other" is the most important step in any encounter. Considering the horse means, first of all, ensuring to avoid making him helpless or turning him into a reactive animal, and ensuring the horse can keep awareness of his body, his own sensations, and inner states. It means learning how to give room to his cognitive abilities and allow him to experience and express his own emotions, attention, curiosity, and inner motivation, both in his life with other horses and in his relationship with humans. This human learning process will consequently bring us to change the activities we will undertake together with a horse, as we'll start to perceive and take into account the horse's point of view.

Here is an example of how you can change your approach from an expectation to a shared experience, while also helping the horse in the understanding of his own environment:

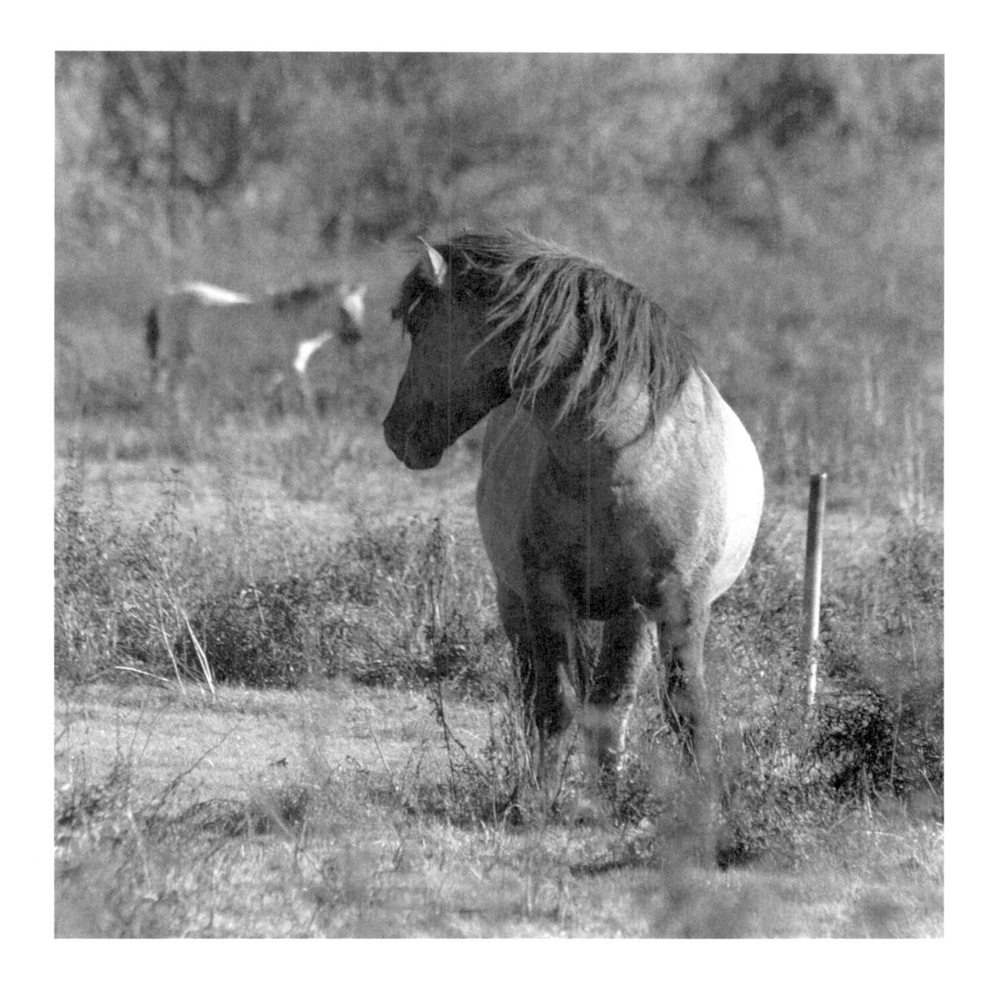

When a horse is being taken out of a field but passes through the gate in a tense way, you can either try to convince him to stay calm, or you can decide to understand that "going out of the gate" could become an experience instead of a necessary obstacle to overcome before you can do the things you planned to do. You can create an experience to allow the horse to get comfortable, and more importantly, create an idea about the gate and the situation around it.

For instance, interacting with the horse inside the field, exploring the gate together, or you going just outside the gate alone while the horse watches you explore a strange bucket, help to reduce all the tension the horse has accumulated by not having been able to explore his surroundings properly. They allow the horse to calm down and recover the serene inner state in which he can elaborate things, understand the gate, and look at the bucket, without needing to put up any resistance. He is able to explore them indirectly and without interference.

▶ *Understanding the "Other" starts with understanding the "Other's" world (how hay smells and feels), allowing the curiosity for the "Other" to grow, before actually meeting him.*

As such, the horse isn't pushed toward his boundaries and the accumulation of tension. This kind of exploring gives him the time—his time—to understand a situation. It changes your perception of experiencing the horse, as well, because instead of projecting your need for a certain activity on the horse, you can start to actually share an experience by perceiving how someone else (the horse) perceives the world.

"It is not what you achieve that is important but how you grow together."
—José De Giorgio-Schoorl

A relationship cannot be developed when it is based on a behavioral outcome that has to be controlled. You only need to create the right context, offer a safe haven in which the horse can have a balanced development, and from which he will himself understand what the best way is to handle a situation. Relationships are made of perceived moments and exchanges, expressions connected to your own inner intention. They are not formed by sequences of automatic behavior, or a continuous pressure of desired outcomes.

Making the Cognitive Horse Visible in Education

Both in the academic world and in other educational programs, people are starting to show an interest in equine perception. This is very

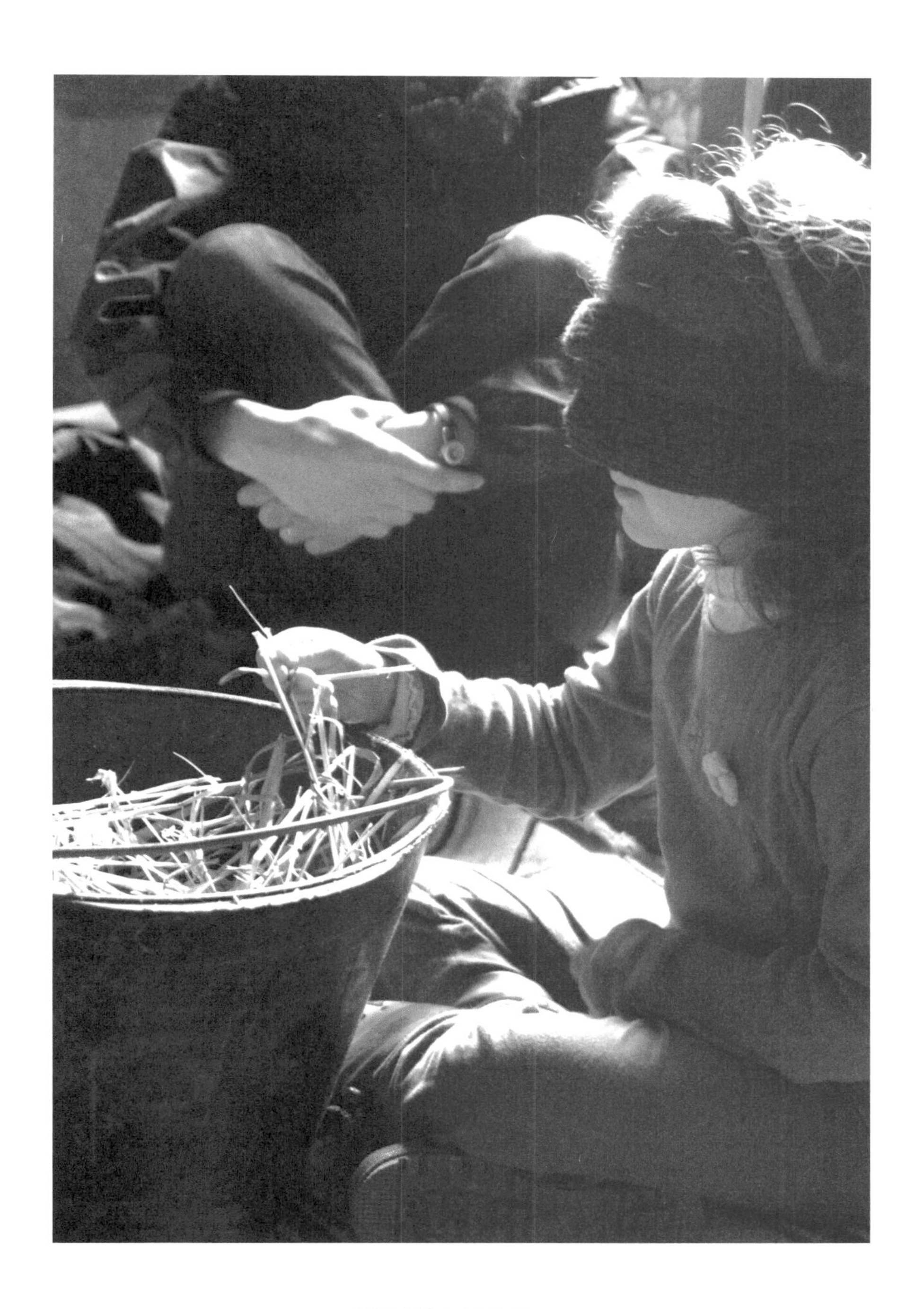

important because in many horse-related institutes, the learning materials used are often influenced and "trapped" by an outdated approach to horse welfare that is more connected to the rider dimension than to the horse dimension.

Training, for instance, which has a huge impact on the socio-cognitive abilities of horses, is intrinsically linked with the instrumentalization (to use merely as a means) of animals. However, these training methods, even the most modern and innovative, are not fitting in a world where a growing awareness for non-human animals is developing. Research about horses should support and encourage the understanding of the horse's intrinsic value, well-being, and quality of life and not from an anthropocentric point of view.

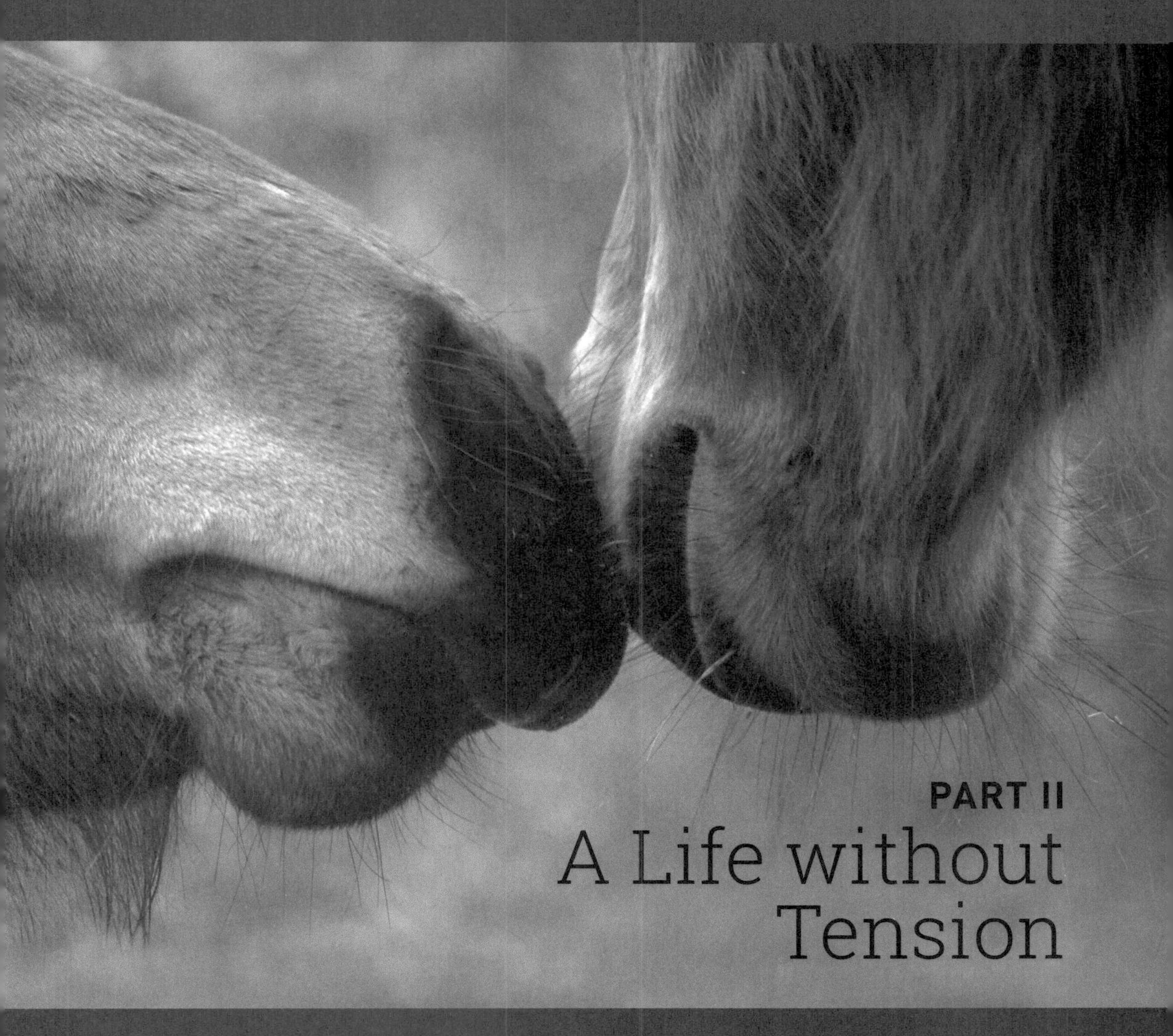

PART II
A Life without Tension

A delicate dialogue of better understanding: no specific goal, just getting to know each other, in a socio-cognitive dimension.

5

The Affiliative Herd

It is early morning in the middle of the summer. The sun is still low, playfully creating long shadows on the ground, while the light seems to unite everything: the blades of grass, the sky, the butterflies, the trees, the shadows, and the eight horses that are standing near each other, eating some hay spread on the ground around them. It is a family group of horses, mostly brothers and sisters, aged from two to nine: a mother, a father, their two-year-old son, and his aunts and uncles. You can hear the sound of their chewing filling the air like a mantra. A four-year-old mare is standing a little farther away, watching people working in the fields, and enjoying the warmth of the first rays of sun on her coat as the air is still cool after the night. One of the males puts a hoof on the hay in front of him to be able to tear some away more easily with his mouth, while another does the same with a branch that has fallen on the ground, tearing off the bark. Two young mares eat strands of hay hanging from each other's mouths, just for the interaction.

Suddenly, one of the mares raises her head and makes a short, soft, but clear nicker, just as one of the males expresses some irritation toward a male beside him, who then decides to distance himself.

The mare foresaw this moment and nickered to ask them to calm down—somewhere between a warning and a reassuring tone.

Then, once this moment has passed, the male who had distanced himself calmly goes back to where he was eating. As he passes in front of the mare, she makes a low, soft sound—the familiar sound horses use to greet each other or to greet a human; the one a mare uses with her foal. Then all continues as it was before, in the same serene atmosphere.

These eight horses live together in a family group, sharing experiences, enjoying life and each other's presence. Leadership and hierarchy are difficult to discern, because they aren't there. The horses form a family. They all watch each other, learn from each other, fine-tune their dialogues, and know each other's particularities. Each one of them takes initiatives, takes the others' individualities into account, and checks the others when something happens. Whether they stand together or graze somewhere individually, they manifest clear affiliative behavior, with radiant and calm attention toward each other and their environment.

We can pick out the following elements from this little episode:

- Even if not directly involved, a horse can foresee the actions of another horse and understand their impact on the rest of the group by reading into situations and understanding the small gestures and inner states of the other horses (as the mare did in this case).
- There is preventive and post-conflict behavior between horses, such as reassuring dynamics and affiliative behavior. In this context, the social dynamics do not define hierarchic relationships but have a bonding purpose.
- Horses use different vocal expressions for different situations.
- For horses, the understanding of a situation (which involves elaborating, gathering, and interpreting information) can be just as important as eating.

Each of these elements is an interesting field of study, both from a relationship point of view and that of equine well-being. However, they are not easily studied if the horse has not had the opportunity to live in a cognitive context with a family-like group. Another hindrance in the study of these elements is our habit of examining a situation with schemes that are related to hierarchy and dominance. We focus on trying to find these rather than being aware of other elements. Also, when we focus on trying to recognize these hierarchical (ranking order) structures, we are often not aware of the fact that we're actually observing unstable situations, with high levels of arousal, and that the social-conflict behavior dynamics being seen are due to the unstable context in which they occur, rather than to the horses involved. We tend to label a horse as the dominant one when that horse could, for example, simply be irritated by the reactive behavior of the other horses. The typical state of arousal that we notice is often due to their living conditions rather than an innate state of being.

▶ *In a family-like group, empathy and shared culture create synchronized movements.*

Another reason why dynamics of conflict are often seen among horses is that the group dynamics these horses experience are rarely born within that group alone. These dynamics don't only depend on that specific group of horses, but also on the context in which that group lives, and the human interaction with every single horse living in that group, part of that group. The fact that they live in contexts that do not respect their needs also means horses gradually lose their socio-cognitive abilities and are no longer able to communicate in more delicate ways.

However, when horses live together in stable semi-family groups, when they are familiar with each other and are not faced with human performance/training pressure, it is easy to see them prevent conflicts, interfere on the rare occasions conflicts do occur, and accompany any conflict with moments of consolatory behavior.

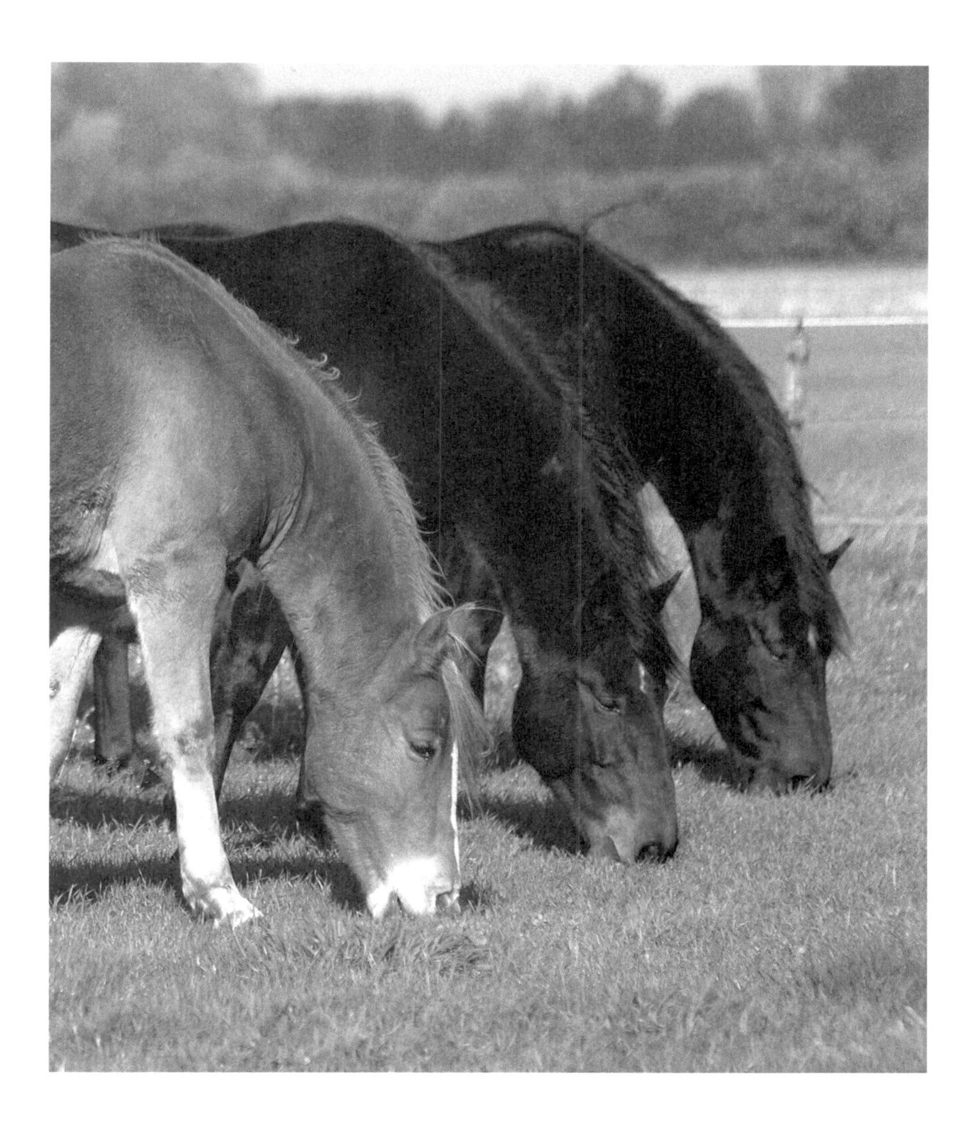

When they live in a natural habitat and family-type groups, horses spend most of their days involved in social dynamics. Even when they are foraging, they are not just foraging but also walking together and being aware of each other's movements, interests, and inner states.

6

The Myth of Equine Hierarchy

The Essence of Horses

Due to the vicious circle of hierarchical focus and our anthropocentric views, there are many elements and details of equine behavior that we fail to see. In fact, we still miss the essential part of the horse—that is, the horse as he is, a sentient and cognitive being, with his own social preferences.

Luckily, these two obstacles are gradually making room for new developments in the fields of ecology, ethology, and evolution. These changes are necessary because even if many people feel there is "more" to the horse and his social behavior than traditionally believed, the strong influence of myths, and the image of the horse as a reactive and unpredictable flight animal, prevail.

Me Tarzan, You Jane

The first question horse people ask themselves when they go to see a new herd is likely to be, "Who is the dominant horse?" Yet, by focusing on this aspect, we immediately create a filter and make it impossible to observe the more subtle social behaviors, all the small gestures, and less visible behaviors that nevertheless have an important cohesive function within the herd.

These gestures can include: observing each other and being aware of the herd's dynamics, looking from a distance while foraging, standing in proximity to each other, separating horses that tend to enter into conflict, smelling each other's noses or flanks to understand certain situations better, and coming to stand close by. Further, horses softly nicker when there is tension between herd members. They are dedicated to all these interactions, which serve to demonstrate understanding and reassurance while reinforcing the role of dialogue within the group.

White Ethology and Black Ethology: Which Side Is Science On?

Ethology, the study of animal behavior, has always represented an important discipline to me. Since I was an adolescent, I've made important decisions in life, dedicated to ethology—a great passion, a study to be explored, to deepen research *for* and *with* animals, not against them.

Today I distinguish two kinds of ethology. First, the "white" one, which aims to understand animal behavior and their perception of the world, to understand how to improve or guarantee their quality of life. Second, the "black" one, which aims to understand animal behavior for anthropocentric purposes like performance and sport.

And I have strived, resolutely and day by day, for a world in which, when we are engaged with animals and their behavior and emotional and mental heritage, it is done without any kind of black ethology—in observation, in interpretation, and in understanding interaction with humans.

We can see the impact of the dominance filter when looking at some of the methods used in groundwork, where a horse is in a round pen and a human is standing in the middle with, or without, a longe line, forcing a horse into movement by gesturing with his arms, believing he is using them as symbols of the leading mare and the pushing stallion. Not only is this not ethical because it doesn't reflect the complex and sophisticated social herd dynamics, but it also brings people to believe that this is actually how horses create dialogue, causing a huge element for miscommunication in the horse-human relationship.

When multiple competitive or conflict behaviors are present, while fewer affiliative and cooperative elements (such as the subtle supportive herd interactions discussed earlier) are exhibited, it is a warning signal, indicating a state of distress within the group. Cooperative and affiliative behaviors are easily observable in groups that live in a permanent social situation. The social stability of the group is an important factor to improve a good quality of life in domestic horses.

▶ *There are many ways to meet.*

Horses do not like conflict. They want to understand social dynamics, watch nuances, and support each other in order to have and preserve a calm environment. They do not busy themselves with ranking but with observing social relationships.

In the horse-human relationship, tricks and treats cannot be used to smooth out and reduce tense behavior. They cannot make it disappear or create in its place an emotionally balanced animal. Our desire for obedience, surrender, and specific reactions makes us cover up behavior and doesn't allow the horse to use his own social skills and inner intentions. Training methods focus on surrender, ignoring the essence of the horse and his social abilities.

Why Lead if What You Really Want Is to Share?

In a reciprocal relationship, there is no need for leadership. All individuals have their intrinsic value, their own strengths and preferences,

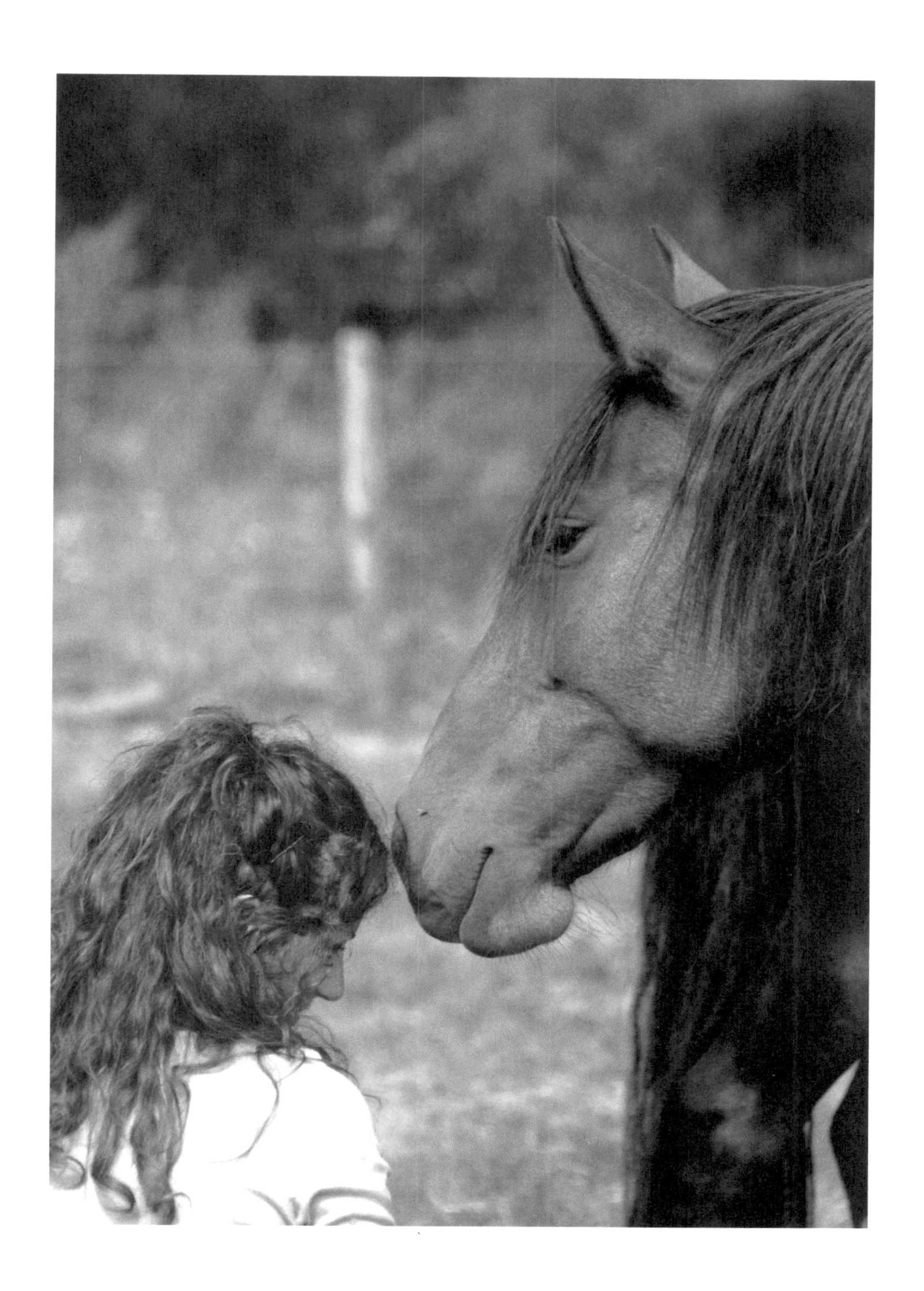

their own unique ways of feeling inspired and motivated. Every relationship is a unique mixture of these elements and when the relationship is what matters the most in us being with someone, whether human or non-human animals, we can learn to become more aware of these elements. In doing so, we create space for a more authentic interaction, for a reciprocal and compassionate dialogue, where both parties can be truly themselves and both individuals feel they can express themselves freely.

In our current coexistence with horses, the following doubts and worries often come up when people start to imagine a reciprocal relationship: Don't we need leadership to be able to go out with a horse? When a horse gets scared, don't we need to guide him? Shouldn't we always try to be in control if something unexpected happens? Isn't it disrespectful when a horse bites us?

What happens is that we so easily cross our own boundaries that we don't recognize how often we take for granted the fact that our equine companions are asked to cross their boundaries, as well. Yet, if we want to improve the horse's quality of life and develop a true relationship, we need to be aware of the more subtle elements of this relationship and take them into account. Only then will both parties feel independently confident and be able to truly enjoy the possibility of undertaking activities *together,* acknowledging that this might mean simply exploring the area outside the paddock. In a shared experience situation, "shared" does not mean that all elements are shared or experienced in the same way. It is about being open and aware of the "Other's" attention and inner state, as well as being willing to share our own. It does not necessarily mean having the same interests and emotions.

"Having an experience" means letting go of any targets we have in mind. When we "lead" it makes us constantly define results, while when we are enjoying a relationship, we enjoy an "experience." If we go to a museum, or take a long walk on the beach with a best friend, we don't worry about who is taking the lead. What is important here is not the target we have in mind, but how we get there and what we experience along the way. It is like a journey to Ithaca: something to treasure, without any hurry to arrive. There is no need for perfection—to have that specific gait, particular movement, or perfect pattern of steps. A relationship with a horse is a precious thing that we should want to treasure every day, caring for the context and the exchange, not for the desired behavioral result.

7

Cognitive Inside

I Was Born a Cognitive Foal

A good example of where the vicious circle can start and misunderstandings begin is the foal and his first encounters with humans. The following is some frequent advice about interacting with a young foal: "Do not let him walk over you, do not let him push you, do not let him bite you, do not let him touch you with his forelegs. Start introducing him as soon as possible to the halter; if not, you will not be able to do it anymore and your foal will grow up spoiled."

If we summarize all the beliefs that exist in the horse world, we would wonder why we should even begin to look for a relationship in the first place!

A foal needs to explore and understand interactions. He has the ability to understand balanced social interactions, and will learn to measure them according to his own cognitive inner state. Horses avoid reactive behaviors if they have the chance to grow up with full awareness of their body and a clear understanding of social dynamics. They do not need a human to control their behavior to teach them their boundaries. Rather, they need a human who will recognize the situation dynamics. For example, if a foal comes up to smell us, it is often found to be "nice." However, we find it very difficult to let an animal simply observe us or smell us, and find out how that feels, how his nose feels, and the soft touch of his whiskers. Instead of sharing that moment, we start touching the foal. By doing this, we interrupt the exploration process and create a higher level of arousal in the foal; we start, for example, to move his head away, which the human then also responds to with his own increase of reactive behavior (enthusiasm or more alertness). The foal then becomes reactive, too, making the human react, and the exchange often ends with the human pushing the foal away. Having lived this experience, the foal is more likely to be in a state of inner conflict the next time he comes to explore.

The art of the interaction is to keep it a cognitive experience: long enough to prevent misunderstandings, short enough to avoid creating confusion. It requires us to make room for a moment of elaboration in which we decentralize ourselves from the active experience, move out of the contact, and give space to the foal's world of perception. If we ignore this, we create a starting point for the foal to gradually lose his mental and emotional balance.

Help! I Have My Own World of Perception

Explorative behaviors are fundamental to preserving cognitive ability. Here is an example to show how equestrian education currently sows the seeds of conflict, thus impacting cognitive ability by stressing the need for anthropocentric control:

A rider decides to take his horse out for a walk. As they go along the path, the horse is observing his environment. Then, on the way, he sees a field full of young calves for the first time. He stops and stands still a short distance before reaching the field to study the situation. This also allows him to maintain a calm inner state and enable the processing of what he is seeing.

Unfortunately, it is at this crucial moment that the rider intervenes.

Due to the prevailing image of the reactive horse that might decide to run away when he sees something strange, and the equestrian principle of always being in control of one's horse, the rider immediately gives leg pressure to "encourage" the horse to walk on. This is almost an automatic reaction from the rider, answering an undesired behavior of the horse instead of understanding the horse's perception.

By trying to push the horse forward and leave the situation, the rider creates a distraction and interruption of the horse's elaboration, which may even cause the horse to react with a flight response as he is unable to keep a cognitive context (for example, by standing still) in which to process that very situation. Instead, the rider should dismount and start observing and exploring the situation with his horse. The rider could share the experience and be a companion.

▶ *Less is more.*

Protagonists of Their Own Lives

To be able to recognize the horse as a cognitive being, the first step is to recognize subjectivity in horses, which is more than simply acknowledging the horse as a sentient living being. As previously explained, recognizing subjectivity in horses has a lot to do with letting go of our tendency to instrumentalize horses.

Roberto Marchesini, author of *Foundations of Zooanthropology,* says: "Subjectivity is the main fulcrum around mentalistic reasoning; it is both the starting point and the aim of the cognitive approach in explaining the human and non-human animal behavioral phenomenon. The fact of having 'subjectivity' means to be interpreters of their own time, or in other words:

- Not to be robots driven by protocols of input and output.
- To be able to create an own experience of the world.
- To be actual protagonists in interactions as free agents and not merely as puppets moved by strings."

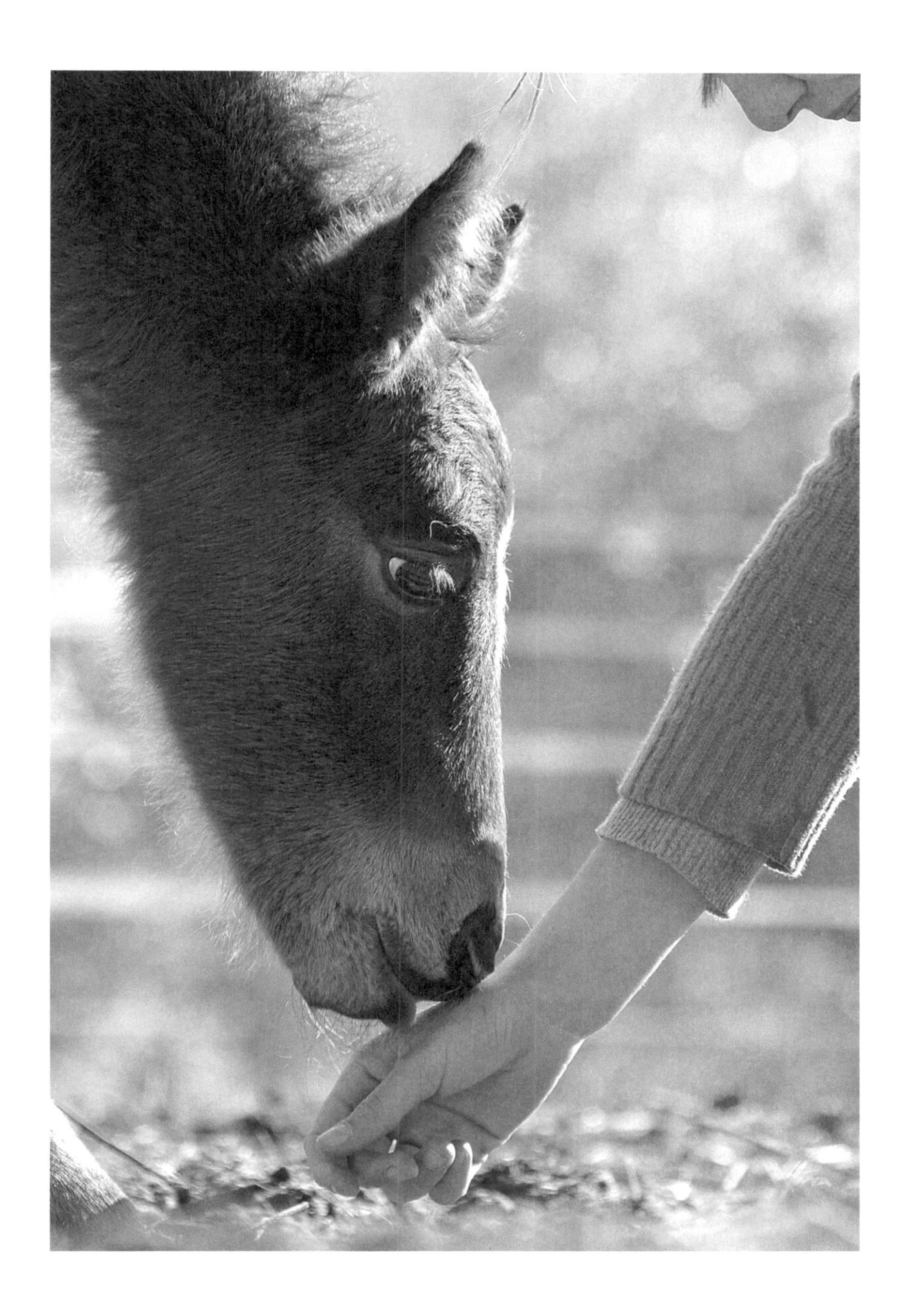

Acknowledging subjectivity can be challenging for many people because it asks us to look at things from a different perspective and make different choices in our relationship with horses. An additional difficulty arises when horses have already been influenced by their training and respond to humans or other horses reactively or with an automatic reaction.

When we are faced with a "problem situation," for instance, when a horse displays what humans define as a "difficult behavior," we tend to follow a linear approach and try to control and change the horse's behavior in order to obtain a "desired outcome."

▶ *Create room for a foal to be the protagonist in his own learning experience.*

Sometimes, we can also get drawn into a vicious circle and increase tension rather than dilute it. For example, when a horse rushes toward us when we enter the paddock, our reaction can increase the horse's excitement and arousal due to the effect of the horse's fast approach. Indeed, by increasing our focus on the horse, our presence becomes a sort of magnetic activator, and both the horse and the human are sucked into a charged interaction, unable to focus on anything else, and the tension just gets higher and higher.

It isn't surprising that these vicious circles that we unknowingly create with our own initial approach, and which, in turn, provoke a reactive behavior on the horse's part, produce situations that encourage us to think in terms of leadership/dominance and conditioning/counter-conditioning—and justify their use.

Aggressive or Confused?

It isn't easy to break through our seeking personal affirmation by establishing hierarchies, because in our society we have been trained to forget how to experience. To be able to share an experience, we need to let go of this urge to seek hierarchies and to create expectations. We need to be able to switch from focusing on our own world of perception, senses, and inner state, to that of the horse. Sharing an experience also

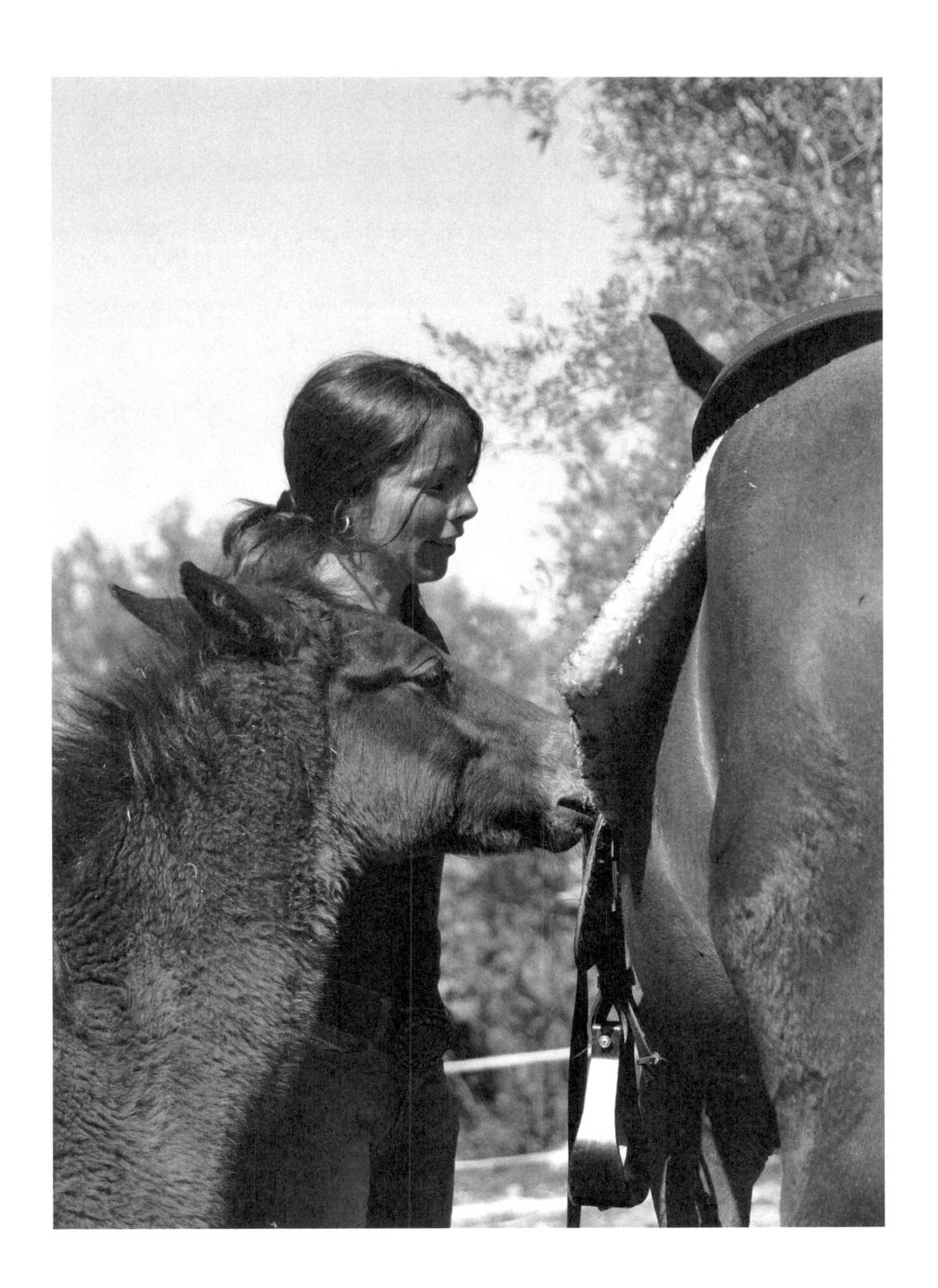

requires a lot of effort on the horse's part, as a life of conditioning has brought him to forget or ignore his senses, and awareness of his feelings, emotions, and intentions. It is a double circle of conditioning and misunderstanding that needs to be broken, but it is worth it.

For some horses and humans, this journey back to their core can be more demanding and, hence, necessary. For instance, horses that have become so confused that they become aggressive, or owners who have done everything with the best of intentions, but realize they don't understand their horses and feel they aren't "meant" for each other—these are situations that are highly emotional and where misunderstanding in the relationship just creates more tension.

The story of Mistral, who came to our rehabilitation center for a year, is an example of these circles of misunderstanding.

When his owner first called us, Mistral was a nine-year-old stallion who was showing increasingly aggressive behavior. The owner loved the horse intensely and had had him since he was a foal, but after using a modern training technique of groundwork, had noticed that her brave stallion had become dangerous, and she was now extremely concerned about the situation.

The first time Francesco met Mistral he found him in a paddock that was surrounded with high wooden fences, a kind of paddock that made you think King Kong must be kept inside. He started by exploring the context outside the paddock. He observed the barn and he smelled the stall where Mistral had lived his whole life and spent most of his days. Then he walked toward the paddock where Mistral went back and forth with extremely reactive movements, expressing his frustration and tension. Francesco waited a while, then when Mistral briefly looked around the paddock to see if there was anything else, Francesco opened the gate and walked in, focusing on exploring the fences and not paying any attention to the stallion. While touching the fence, he wondered if it could really keep something the size of

King Kong inside. Then he explored the sand looking for prints, but still without focusing on Mistral who was beginning to pay attention to Francesco's movements, expecting an approach from him. Eventually, Mistral ran toward Francesco, reacting to his own expectations, but Francesco just continued his exploration. Mistral, intrigued by this strange presence, became investigative himself: he began to smell Francesco's shoulders, legs, and came to explore the fences with him. From being in a reactive state, he changed in that moment into a cognitive and curious presence.

A few weeks later, Mistral came to live in our rehabilitation center with our band of equine bachelors, where he finally found a socio-cognitive context in which he could learn how to socialize with others in an affiliative way, without any pressure or dominance episodes. He became himself again, sensitive and curious toward other horses and humans. Today, he lives in a social dimension enjoying his interactions with other horses and his human companion.

8

The Mental Cage of Conditioning

Nature Is Not Negative

It is still commonly believed that, in nature, dynamics among social animals are governed by dominance hierarchies. Even in the scientific world, we often hear about the dominance hierarchy of social animals, and several decades ago, classical ethology defined this model of interpretation to describe intra-species dynamics.

The concept of leadership and alpha individuals in social animals was emphasized by studies that were done in the 1940s about the social dynamics of wolves. The studies were conducted in an artificial environment where the social context was missing: The wolves that were brought together for the research often came from different wolf packs, which meant that the more sophisticated dialogues relating to family relationships were nonexistent. Thus, it seemed that the wolves were organized in pecking orders in which they would fight and compete strongly for a higher ranking.

In the last 30 years, this model of interpretation has been repeatedly questioned by scientists and philosophers, making room for different views about animal behavior and social dynamics. Interactions need to be interpreted within their complex social context: We should not offer an interpretation basing ourselves on a one-to-one interaction that is isolated from the dynamics of the whole social context; similarly, interactions should not be analyzed in a very limited time span, where pre- and post-interactions are not included.

If we look, for example, at a pack of wolves in its natural habitat and configuration, we can observe a family group where dynamics are nuanced and where many interactions are based on the reciprocal development of skills and social abilities. They share experiences to broaden behavioral expressions and become more agile in the different interactions with the individuals of that family pack. They learn how to take each other into account, from understanding each other's individual ways of expression. It is possible to see that every wolf has different emotional and cognitive skills in a social organization. Dominance behaviors are less frequent and not used to improve or establish relationships, but to handle a certain situation. Today, new insights have changed the way we look at group dynamics, but in the meantime, this hierarchy myth has been used to explain the social dynamics of other animals as well as the human-animal interaction.

It is similar in the equestrian world, where all the main traditions and training techniques seek discipline, human control, and the horse's submission. As a result, although people might have been very skilled in empathic understanding and affiliative behavior, they learn to lead and even risk losing these important social abilities for the incorrect sake of dominating an animal.

Because one hears the "alpha mare" mantra, over and over again and is told about the supposed strict hierarchies and punishments in nature, it is difficult to be objective when we observe horses' reactions toward man. To make it more complicated, training techniques are sometimes labeled "natural" although they have little to do with nature. If we look, for example, at the natural horsemanship methods, the superficial eye might be satisfied that the horse doesn't seem to be physically harassed, but the mental abuse is very intense, easier to ignore, and much more difficult to heal. The only thing that happens "naturally" if one is continually and repeatedly pressured and frightened, is in the end, that "someone" probably ends up doing what we want. Using fear as a way of creating yet another reactive response in any living being is both unethical and highly activates the reactive stimulus responses again, as do all other anthropocentric training methods.

▶ *Change perspective; follow the horse.*

The following anecdote refers to a particular social moment we observed between stallions that shows how inappropriate the strict ranking regulations are.

During one of our visits to a group of horses living in semi-feral conditions in the south of the Netherlands, we were walking along the main road situated just outside the nature reserve. As it is slightly higher up, we had a good view over the area. There, in the reserve, lived two groups of horses: a herd of several mares with a stallion, and a small group of four young bachelor males. We were watching the bachelors who were walking near a pool when a fifth horse suddenly appeared. At first we thought we hadn't counted well, but using the binoculars, we recognized the stallion of the harem. He had temporarily left his herd of mares to go and look for the nearby bachelor group. What we then saw had nothing to do with dominance or the affirmation of positions: it was an intense social contact, a calm interaction of greetings with some elements of play and a social cognitive exchange. It lasted about 20 minutes. They even grazed together for a moment before the stallion returned to his herd.

Nature is not negative. In fact, if we examine them more closely, we notice that the explanations humans find in nature to justify their approach to horses (especially when it comes to "inappropriate

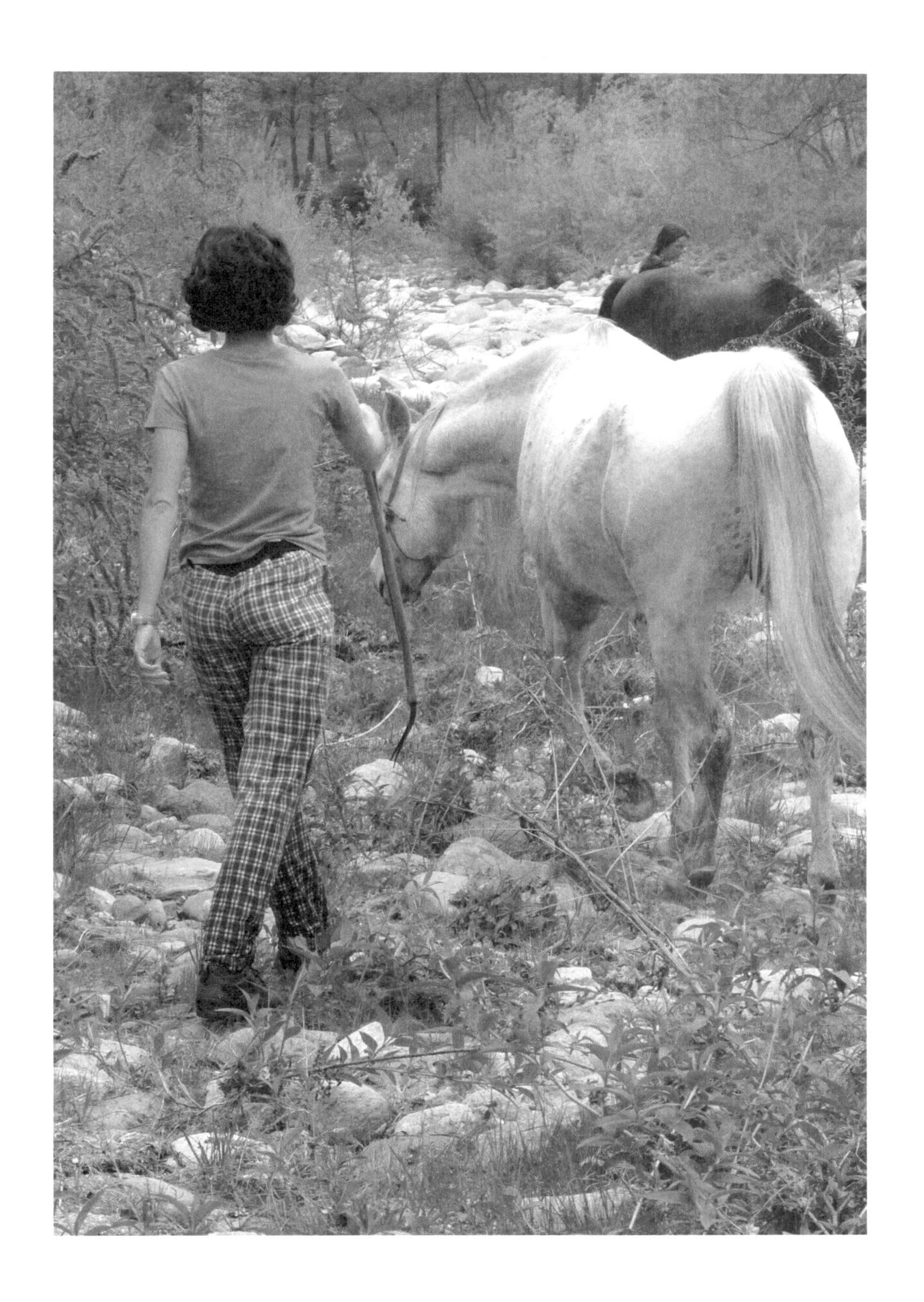

behavior") are linked and bound to our filtered perceptions. We blindly overlook the patience, acceptance, and room for self-expression that horses show in a natural setting. Our preconceptions prevent us from seeing that horses are social animals that are able to develop a sophisticated social dialogue, both within their own species and with other species (including humans), that is not based on mistrust, tension, or competition.

Not only does this deep misunderstanding not honor the social intelligence of the horse, but it also has a negative impact on the relationship with implications on the horse's welfare and well-being. For example, we desperately want our horses to be engaged in their interactions with us but do not leave them the autonomy to do so. We don't take the time to enjoy a balanced relationship and often bring tension by continuously requiring inputs and reactions, seeking our own satisfaction and hoping to reach our own objectives. Yet, a horse needs to be able to be self-directed and have self-awareness in order to be "engaged" in a relationship.

Often we want to create a balanced relationship but set up a situation that is not balanced from the outset. For instance, the horse may find himself in an awkward situation (for example, social isolation during the first training encounters), or we may apply methods that are based on operant conditioning, both of which drastically reduce the possibility for spontaneous behaviors.

The next problem that occurs is that the reactive behaviors that develop are then often mistaken for free choices. Yet, a horse running toward a person in a paddock with food expectations, or a horse following you in a round pen without wearing a halter, are not free choices at all. These horses merely display macro behaviors that please us from an anthropocentric point of view, while also showing micro signals of internal conflict, frustration, or apathetic behaviors.

The fascination for behavioral training methods comes from the illusory sensation of control that they provide as they enable us to verify the progress of training as if we were trying to optimize a chain process. Being able to measure the behavioral response as soon as the human gives a stimulus makes it possible for the human to judge whether there is a good result or not, while keeping an analytic distance from the animal. Clearly, in this kind of interaction and with this objective in mind, it is easy to ignore the animal's social and cognitive skills, as well as his emotions, identity, inner motivation, perception of the world, and ability for self-expression. One ends up with a distorted vision of horse emotions. As an example, just think of all the images we see that depict horses in agonistic (conflicting) activities with a trainer ultimately "winning" an "argument" over a horse's behavior. Many people see this as the horse thinking through and making a choice, when in fact he is distressed. The following anecdote is about a zooanthropologic consult for a 12-year-old mare.

Venice was cognitive inside, but she had repeatedly experienced pressure from groundwork techniques for a long period of time, which had created a lot of resistance and automatisms (spontaneous reactive behavior) in her. Although these exercises had been interrupted for months when we met her, and she had supposedly been "free" to act and behave as she wanted, her reactive and schematic behavior had not gone away and would ignite at the slightest gesture or movement. In her case, the way forward was to deconstruct habits by creating an experience in which she could break these behavioristic schemes.

The activities would take place in her usual paddock, and depended on how Venice perceived our presence. Allowing her to break her automatic reactions would mean that she had to be able to let go of her expectations toward human interaction. Allowing her to look at humans with curiosity again so that her cognitive state could become more present, she could be relaxed and herself, interacting with her human companion.

Offering objects to explore did not intrigue Venice, she simply waited for a training gesture and remained in her tensed and reactive automatism. So Francesco started to walk in a strange way, like a drunken man: imprecise movements, without objective, strange and unknown to Venice, enabling her to begin to break her expectations and previous mindset. She began to follow him with her gaze and visually explore the different movements. When he dropped on the ground, like a drunken man, she actually came to smell him. This was

The Cognitive Dog

From reactive energy to cognitive energy: here's an experience where reactive energy is transformed into a cognitive flow.

What *is* part of the experience:

- A human: calm, aware, present in the moment
- An H-harness
- A 30-foot line
- A natural environment
- Imprecision

What is *not* part of the experience:

- No human with expectations, goals, objectives, or a result-driven mindset
- No collar (any type of collar)
- No jerking
- No food whatsoever, not as reinforcement, nor as target
- No commands (sit, stay, or wait)
- No perfection, no precision

The experience starts with the human making contact with the outside, in the forest or woods, absorbing the environment with all senses, while the dog follows—making contact in his own way.

The human stops and breathes in deeply, his hands touch the ground, without any predefined goals, just living the moment; the dog also explores, the long, loose line gets rubbed in the soft ground and starts blending in with the earth, with the human making sure not to let it get stuck between the low branches. From time to *her first genuine approach for a long time. José then began to help Venice's human companion to deconstruct her own habits, as well.*

From Control Back to Contact

Humans have divided a horse's life into various phases and have established in detail what the horse should learn in each phase: handling, haltering, walking, wearing a saddle. We precisely define what and

time, the human stops to dig a hole between the roots of some of the trees; the dog approaches every now and then, intrigued by this strange human activity. During these moments of interaction, the human takes the line off the harness, checks physically, and calmly attaches the snap again. They arrive at a pond. The human sits on the shore while the dog starts to explore the waterline, moving in the water, captivated by the sight of dragonflies flying just above it.

The line gets wet and covered with mud. The human takes off his shoes, pulls up his jeans, and starts to explore the water plants, followed by the dog in the shallow water. They seem to search for something together, perhaps traces of otters. The dog becomes increasingly centered, centering himself, in dialogue with the environment, and transforming his reactive energy in a social-emotional, cognitive one, in greater contact with himself, with the environment and with the human.

Then traces of deer appear: the human and the dog sniff together, they feel together, and they touch them together. They return to the village, the line still lingers on the ground between them, dirty with experience. The dog walks calmly, not tired, and he continues to explore with the same intention on his way back.

Facilitating calm does not mean tiring an animal, whether two-legged or four, or teaching him how he should behave. It means giving him an experience in which he can center himself, on an emotional-cognitive level, with an energy that is always in there, and that allows him to become connected with himself.

when the horse should learn and expect it to be done without resistance. To meet all these requirements, training methods are applied, aiming to teach a precise behavior. By focusing on this result, we also slowly and often unknowingly train ourselves to ignore the contact moments as they do not fit into the protocol.

For example, when someone is working with a horse (from the ground or in the saddle) and something happens outside the working area that draws the horse's attention so that the horse stops to listen or look at it, the trainer's most common reaction is to point out that the horse has lost his attention, focus, and concentration. This is, of course, a very strange way of looking at things because in that moment, the horse actually regained attention, focus, and concentration toward the world around him, which he should be in contact with. It is that world he returns to whenever the work is done. We think the horse should shut down every connection he has with the rest of his environment the moment we start an activity with him. Yet, once we get the horse to do this, to focus exclusively on us, we have, in fact, trained both the horse and ourselves to ignore and gradually forget how to be in contact with the world.

▶ *A family: a father, mother, and their daughter.*

The tension that arises from training practices is often due to a lack of awareness of mental pressures, which is, in turn, linked to our lack of recognition of a horse's mental abilities. Unfortunately, the more micro-tensions we create and social skills we ignore, the greater the repercussions on social dynamics (in the horse's interaction with us and with his herd). Some horses become so numb that they can no longer read another horse's signals; some are so stressed that they create irritation in others; or they are so irritated that they redirect their tension toward other herd members to get it out of their system, and in doing so, leave the entire herd in an overall state of tension.

We must remember that, in the wild, a group of horses is first of all a family, where relationships are crucial. It is not a military base,

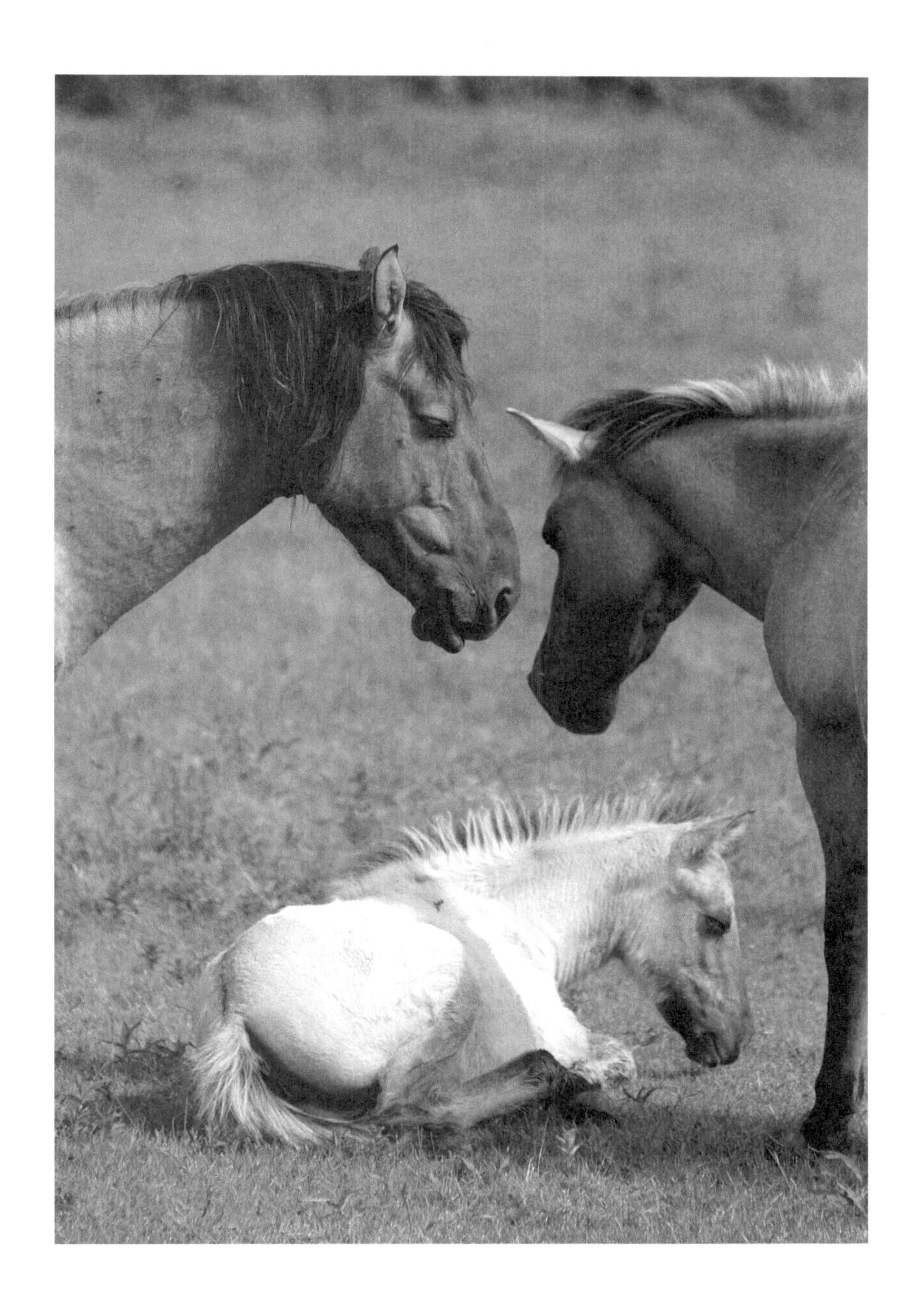

where mechanisms of control, hierarchy, and leadership define interactions. It is a social environment that involves curiosity, empathy, social dynamics, affiliative behavior, and the desire to maintain a calm cognitive context in which each individual can elaborate dynamics without encountering defensive attitudes. It is impossible to understand horse life if we don't try to understand equine cooperative behaviors, as almost all equine social behaviors are affiliative and cooperative, whereas competitive behaviors constitute only a small part of natural social dynamics.

In the horse-human interaction, if we want to learn from natural dynamics, where the horse interacts with others in a social context, we need to understand affiliation, as well.

Affiliative behaviors play a role in social dynamics and are present in many social species, such as primates, wolves, ravens, horses, and others. Alleviation behavior, which is one of these social dynamic functions, is used to reduce distress in other individuals, as well as in the social group as a whole. They can be found in family groups of horses, as well as in family-like permanent groups. For instance, when a horse shows some element of distress—for example, colic pains—the other horses come to stand still around him, for consolation and protection. In doing so, they reduce distress both in the individual and in the group.

Family, family-like, and permanent relationships are fundamental for the expression of these affiliative behaviors. In a recent pilot study made at Learning Animals (www.learning-animals.org), some important elements about social cognition were analyzed. This study introduced an unknown object to a family group of horses in semi-feral conditions, as well as a family-like group of domestic horses and a non-permanent group of domestic horses. It then compared the exploratory process of each group, taking into account the behavior dynamics of each from the moment herd members noticed the object to the initial point of distraction that interrupted their explorative process. Comparing the results indicated interesting differences between the groups, and the results seemed to indicate that group stability, in which individuals take each other into account to avoid tension, allows a better exploratory process and, consequently, a better cognitive experience.

Food Reward? No Thanks. I'm on a Cognitive Diet!

Over the last decades, there has been increasing awareness of animal welfare, as well as a desire to work differently with animals to avoid invasive training techniques. Within these developments, behavioristic learning theory concerning operant conditioning has been used to explain horse behavior. Yet, whether talking about negative or positive reinforcement, operant conditioning has a severe impact on the horse, physically, mentally, and/or emotionally. The simplicity of the learning theory and the possibility to translate it into a set of rules you can follow and a standard by which you can look at a horse, has given it enormous popularity, thus leaving social learning, latent learning, and other cognitive aspects unexplored or even unknown. Its popularity has even been favored linguistically due to the use of the term "positive" (as in positive reinforcement) because it satisfies what we humans think is the maximum we can do for somebody: give him a premium.

When operant conditioning is applied in practice, especially after a horse has shown behavior difficulties, the results seem almost magical to the unprepared eye. Horses effectively seem to learn new behaviors quickly. This responds to the trainers' and owners' desire to keep things under control, and perfectly meets our need to reassure ourselves we have a horse that we can take care of and that will not cause problems. The horse seems to be a "fast learner." However, this mechanical and linear method risks damaging a horse's ability to express himself and his cognitive ability to create his own understanding of a given situation. Psychologists use "learned helplessness" to describe situations when humans or animals lose their capacity to respond to situations even when they have the opportunity to do so—as was the case of Calisto (see below) who didn't move away from things that frightened him. This tendency to behave helplessly is usually caused by the desire to avoid unpleasant circumstances or to gain positive rewards.

> *From one of our students in applied equine zooanthropology, Calisto arrived to me at age three and had practically no experience with people. I had just discovered a training method based on positive reinforcement and thought this would be a nice, friendly method to start working with this young horse. Although the results came fast and I liked them, something didn't feel right.*
>
> *Growing up, he didn't protest when I started riding. There was no flight attitude, he didn't buck, he actually did everything I asked him. As with hoof care, trailer loading, riding out with or without other horses, he was obedient and never caused any problem. But he always had tensed lips. Despite the calm, step-by-step training, and the apparently good results, he showed distrust, even fear with objects near his body. Brushes, the saddle blanket, farrier tools, anything. He wouldn't react on it, but I could see it, I could sense it, and it made me sad. That is how I became interested in understanding more about "the cognitive horse."*

Because they reinforce linear reactions by asking for a precise reaction that is independent from the actual situation the horse is in, operant conditioning and the mechanical training derived from it (whether applying negative or positive reinforcement) disrupts a horse's problem-solving ability, his ability to be creative, and his ability to deal with changing circumstances. The animal is consequently trained, simultaneously, to ignore and inhibit his capacity to create a sound understanding of his environment.

In today's social media, there are countless examples of situations where food rewards are used in interaction with all kinds of animals. Dolphins, dogs, horses, cats, rabbits, zebras, tigers, and many others undergo this kind of conditioning. It might look innocent, but it has a direct impact on their limbic system (comprised of brain structures that are involved in emotions).

We can understand the severity of this impact by looking, for example, at the importance of the senses for horses, for their well-being in general and, more specifically, in their interaction with humans. If we want to improve our understanding of horses and our interaction with them, we need to be aware of how they create their own experience and leave the horse the freedom to do so.

Horses use their olfactory system to process information coming from odors. They explore and smell in order to be connected with their environment and improve their understanding of it. For this reason, when working with horses, we must learn to be aware of how the horse uses his senses, trying to notice and understand when the horse is interested or focusing on something with his senses. It could be anything! Something on the ground, a fence, something in the air....

Some horses (like many humans!) are no longer used to using their sense of smell to improve their understanding of a situation, and as a result, miss important information that could otherwise be reassuring. This "not smelling" is due to constantly overlooking their needs in their interaction with man. When they want to stop to smell along a path, we ask them to continue walking; when they want to take in the smells of an unknown arena, we ask them to start "working," for example.

This problem is accentuated further if horses get used to food premium rewards. By being trained to focus on food, their response is stimulated in the limbic system, and the possibility of remaining calm and explorative is almost entirely taken away. They create a strong association between anything interesting to explore and the possibility of food. Of course, the olfactory system is still working, but from a reactive inner state, with the expectation of finding food, instead of simply processing information from an object. A horse that is smelling with food expectations is easily recognizable: his nostrils pass quickly and mechanically without taking in his surroundings, his breath is superficial, and his nose immediately touches a human's arm or object without first pausing to elaborate the information from a distance or, after slow intense breathing, stopping at a whisker's distance, taking in all that the moment is telling his perception, to take time to build his own map of the situation. We are not used to paying attention to these kinds of details. We might never know what information the horse is getting, but we can learn to recognize his attention and signs of his elaboration.

▶ *What's in a nose? Everything—nuances, expressions, interest, attention, dialogue.*

Food premiums also have an immediate impact on daily activities. For example, when horses in shared pastures start perceiving man as mere food dispensers, the human presence will immediately trigger food expectations and, consequently, tension in the entire group. This is something we need to take responsibility for instead of trying to correct the behavioral consequences (horses become insistent or even irritated when looking for food), which we caused by using food premiums in the first place.

Can't Buy Me Love

We often feel the urge to reward because we forget how to live in the moment. The reward becomes a substitute for actually sharing an experience born from an intrinsic interest. Yet, it is from that interest that an authentic relationship can be developed.

Living a calm, interesting life doesn't need a premium. Life itself should give satisfaction. We live often totally unconnected with ourselves, trying frantically to find contact with the horse, using all kinds of techniques. By offering a premium, we don't give the horse the possibility to relate to us, congruent and in line with himself.

We need to be aware of the fact that when we give food rewards to horses, we create such a strong magnet that we reduce their ability for free expression. Positive reinforcement is a form of operant conditioning that falls within the behaviorist framework. Today, it is high time for

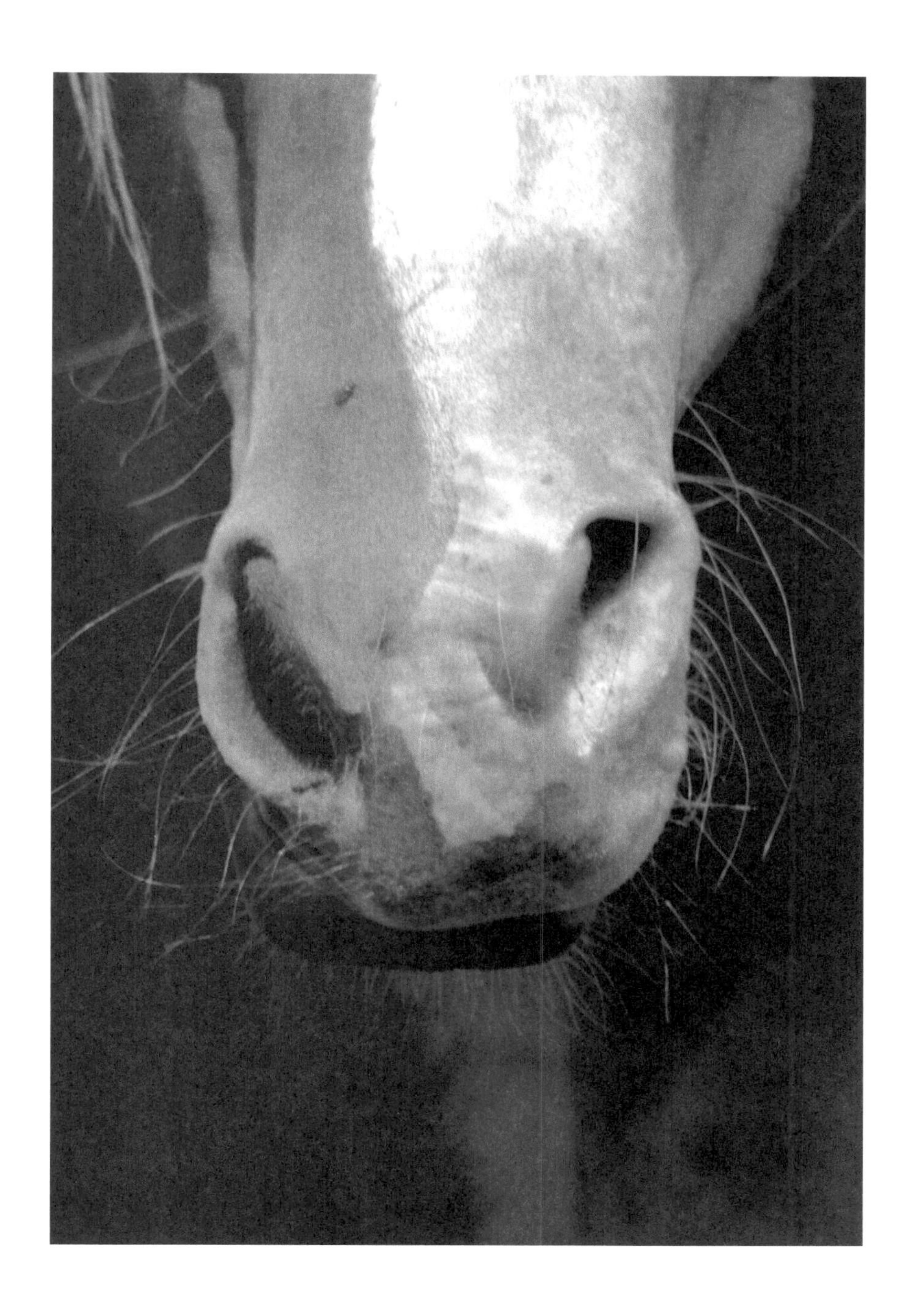

such an approach to human interaction with animals to be thoroughly questioned. Behaviorism completely disregards animals' mental elaboration, emotions, and internal state.

▶ *Everyone and everything can be part of a learning experience.*

Modern training methods and most horse-human interactions are based on the deterministic (that proposes all behavior is caused by preceding factors and thus predictable) and reductionist (the practice of simplifying a complex idea, issue, or condition) approach of operant conditioning as people's minds are still set on the anthropocentric view of animals. They are attracted by the possibility of being able to optimize results, causing methods to talk about seeing the animal as a subject, working on a relationship, on dialogue, trust and togetherness, while in the approach there is still no real understanding of what every single one of these statements means from the horse's point of view. The methods describe a horse as being "free" when working without the use of tack or other instruments, like tigers tamed in a circus. However, you don't need a whip or cookies when you look for dialogue. These methods combine training, taming, breaking, whispering, desensitizing, and other typical training terminology and practices, but always remain unaware of the horse's socio-cognitive ability for developing a relationship with an "Other."

"Freedom to have self-esteem, to make decisions for oneself and to express oneself—that is an inner freedom that will preserve and sustain a healthy body and a healthy mind."
—Francesco De Giorgio

Quality of life and freedom of the mind correspond to other cultural, ethical, practical, and scientific principles that start with looking at the horse as a socio-cognitive being, equally able and engaged in creating his own world of experiences.

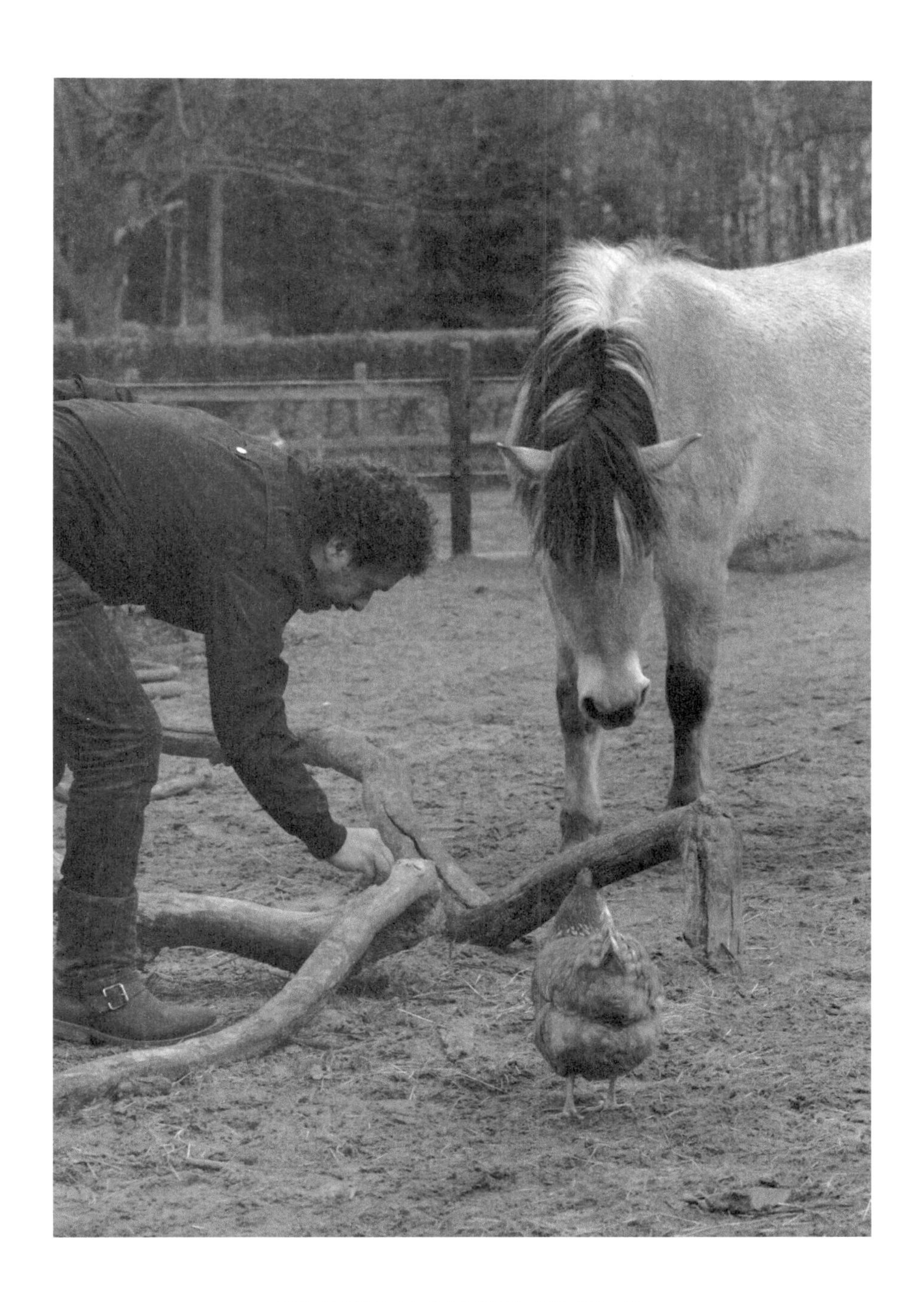

Relaxation and Inner Motivation

One of the more important characteristics of taking into account the cognitive-zooanthropologic model is the mental and physical relaxation of both the horse and human in their interaction. This is very different from operant conditioning (using positive or negative reinforcements), which tends to reduce the possibility of mental flexibility by only allowing linear associations. In that case, a horse's natural cognitive capacities and ability to interpret a situation are reduced, making the horse more dependent on humans and less capable of creating his own understanding. However, a horse should have the right to feel balanced and confident with himself at all times.

When a cognitive horse explores something new, an unknown object for instance, we can easily observe welfare signals such as relaxation, pleasure, and satisfaction. These behavioral signals are a reflection of balanced mental and physical states. Family groups of horses know how to approach situations without creating panic or tension. They know how to live together and communicate with each other while preserving their self-expression and the possibility to interact with their surroundings in a cognitive way.

Cognitive horses—or in other words, horses that have had the opportunity to express their instinctive cognitive potential from birth and have grown up in a socio-cognitive context without performance pressures—like to investigate things. Investigating is part of their evolutionary heritage and experience, and this should be possible for all horses.

Today, the young horse called Calisto is starting to show signs of curiosity. A new learning process has begun, and it is as if he sees and perceives things for the first time: the halter, grooming or hoof-trimming tools, humans, anything. This is a process of rediscovery. Just because we are looking at something doesn't mean we are really seeing it; this applies to horses, as well as humans.

Learn to Learn (Outside the Cage)

The cognitive-zooanthropologic perspective completely revolutionizes the linear schematic stimulus-response tendency of operant conditioning typically applied in horse training. In horse-human interactions, operant conditioning has a linear "one-to-one" structure.

In this cognitive paradigm, we talk about a non-linear "infinity-to-infinity" dimension as everything around us can play a role in the experience and we can never know, precisely, what will be part of the experience. For example, we may be walking up to a horse in a paddock with a halter, when another horse comes to smell it. Creating room for that experience to happen might arouse curiosity in the first horse who comes closer to observe, and maybe even a third horse, who usually tends to keep his distance from the others, comes to smell the halter, too. Those few minutes, lived fully, bring more than three hours of training.

Balanced movements, concentration, and the possibility to look at humans and each other from a different perspective give horses all the necessary elements to find their own balanced (mental and physical) experience. Working this way helps to channel away all the micro-tensions most horses have incorporated because of their coexistence with humans.

The Latin phrase *Beati monoculi in terra caecorum* ("In the land of the blind, the one-eyed man is a king") helps us understand how much more we have to learn from horses in a non-linear dimension. To be able to learn from the horse and take into account his intentions and perception, we must be able to look at him with both eyes open, which metaphorically means with more openness. To be able to think in terms of infinite possibilities and see with both eyes, we need to break the walls set up by the circus of operant conditioning in the minds of humans and animals alike. This is the real ethical challenge for the coming years.

According to the cognitive-zooanthropologic model, the interface of the mind is not a mere exposure to the world through the horizon of sensory sensitivity, but also being proactive and having an inquiring mind with regard to the world. We could say with Heidegger, extending it beyond the human, that the mind is "creator of worlds" *(Schopfer der Welten)*. If we consider the horse's mind a "creator of worlds," it becomes indisputable that operant conditioning reduces it by its linear and mechanical qualities. The creation of worlds belongs, on the contrary, to the horse's cognitive, emotional, affective, and social dimensions.

This approach, obviously, also requires a strong awareness of our own socio-cognitive abilities.

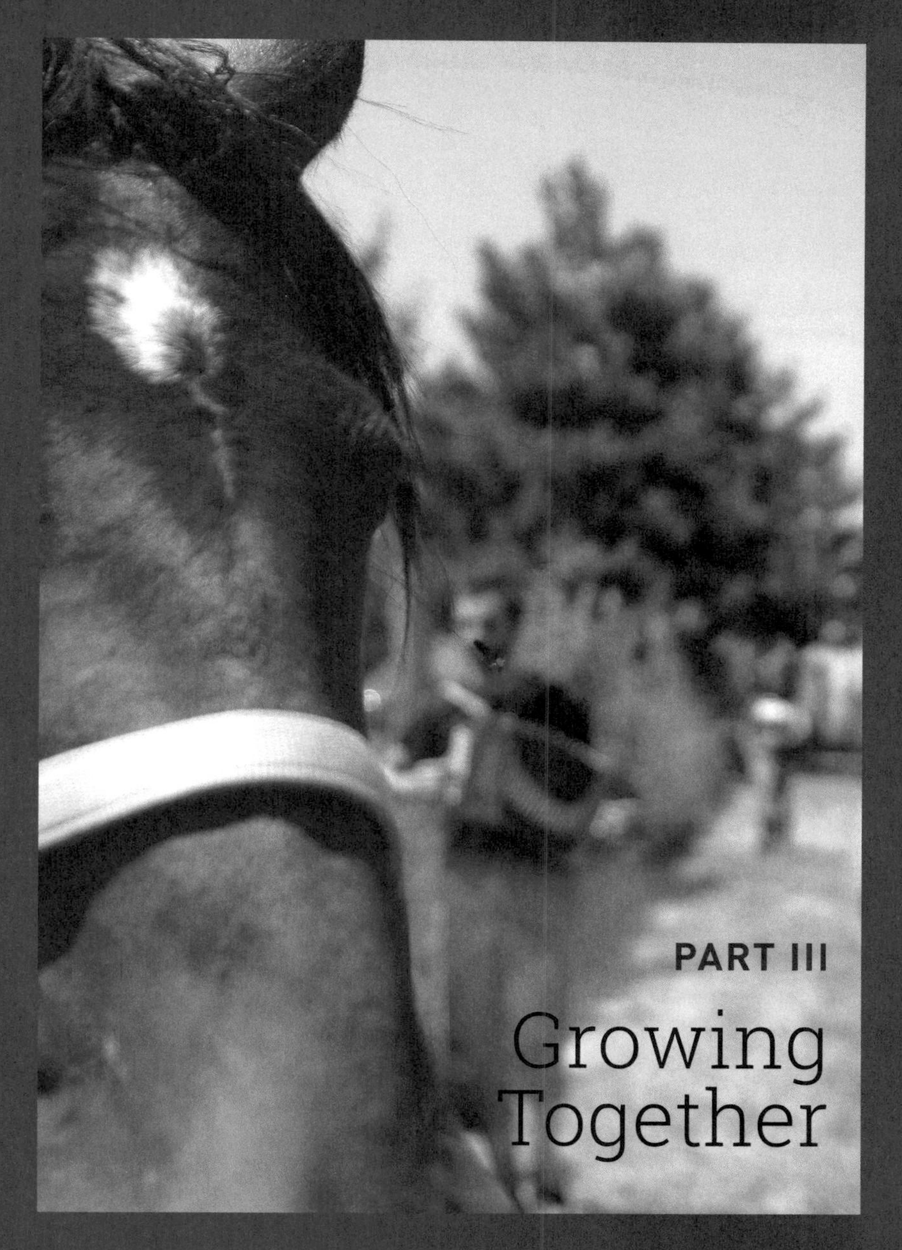

PART III
Growing Together

The sound of music! Imagination is important to broaden horizons and find inspiring situations that facilitate a shared experience.

9

Finding Ground for Dialogue

Marea was born in a herd of horses that live in the hills to the north of Rome. When she was two years old, she was taken out of the herd by cattlemen as she was supposed to have a destiny as a working horse, a "cavallo buttero" as they call them in Italy. However, the traditional training they exposed her to didn't go as expected: the brand marks that were made on both her flanks amplified her anger and defenses, to the point that they decided to interrupt her training and take her back to the mountain to join the herd again. But, by that time, she was a bit lost inside. Being so very young, she was completely puzzled about what these life experiences meant and what she should learn from them.

We met Marea ourselves a year later, when we were visiting her herd in which the mothers of three of our own horses lived. By then, she had decided not to look for contact, not with humans and not with the other horses. Her body was tense and rigid, and she kept her distance from the others. Yet, when we were not looking straight at her, she would glimpse us from under her forelock with some kind of curiosity and attraction. She probably noticed something in our movements and attention that was different from all the things she had perceived in humans until then. We asked the cattlemen to let her go and allow her to come with us, away to another dimension where she could recover from her first confusing encounters with humans.

After another couple of visits, we brought her to join our herd of horses in the Sabina hills, where two of her younger brothers and a younger sister were already living. They had come the previous year, before any training or invasive human intervention.

Marea's defensive behavior and her decision not to follow her intrinsic curiosity made it not very easy to find ways that would allow her to get to know the other horses, let alone us. However, by giving her all the space she needed, and continuing to create experiences with her family members around her, that same glimpse of curiosity could be seen every so often. Then, one day, a situation arose between her and the other horses, and when we came closer to see how she was doing, she very gently bit a part of our clothing, which was clearly a sign that she was trying to make contact and express something from inside. Very carefully, she had found the courage to express something, to see if we would hear her, to see if her expression wouldn't be ignored, or worse, punished (as had happened before). It was a small opening toward the possibility of finding ground for dialogue.

That was the first time she had dared to truly express herself again—following her inner awareness rather than just reacting. But her rehabilitation wasn't easy as her first human experiences hadn't left her with a positive opinion of human interaction. It is usually very difficult for humans to accept that these responses, easily seen as negative, are not personal, but related to what a horse has experienced previously. She had to be given the opportunity to experience new situations and realize, over and over again, that different relationships are possible.

Discovering that she could express some of her inner tension was necessary so that she could get all the resistance she felt out of her system. It also enabled her to find the confidence and self-centeredness she needed to be able to listen to her own intention and motivation and explore the possibilities of establishing a cognitive dialogue with others, so different from the stimulus-response actions in reactive situations—a dialogue based on, and allowing the exploration of, contact-oriented feelings and behavior.

▶ Discovery is often where you don't expect it.

If, instead, she had been gradually exposed to human interaction aiming to desensitize her, she wouldn't have been able to look for contact—she would simply have grown accustomed and accepting of certain interactions. We cannot decide for someone else about when they will be able to feel safe again and stop defensive behavior. It is impossible to know when horses will feel safe again in their interactions with others, or when they will feel strong enough to be able to listen to their own inner self, instead of being in a state of constant alertness, ready to resist whatever might come their way.

Consequently, Marea would just observe and "be" among the other horses, looking for her own experience and understanding of what was happening around her, and never crossing the boundaries of that small space in which she felt safe and comfortable in that moment of time.

After an intense journey of reciprocal observation, studying of interactions, and fine-tuning of expressions, she opened up to the other horses, started to take initiative, and even started to mix in when we were doing exploratory activities with the other horses. She discovered and rediscovered objects like the halter, and she started to explore us, gently, and from a profound state of awareness and newly found curiosity.

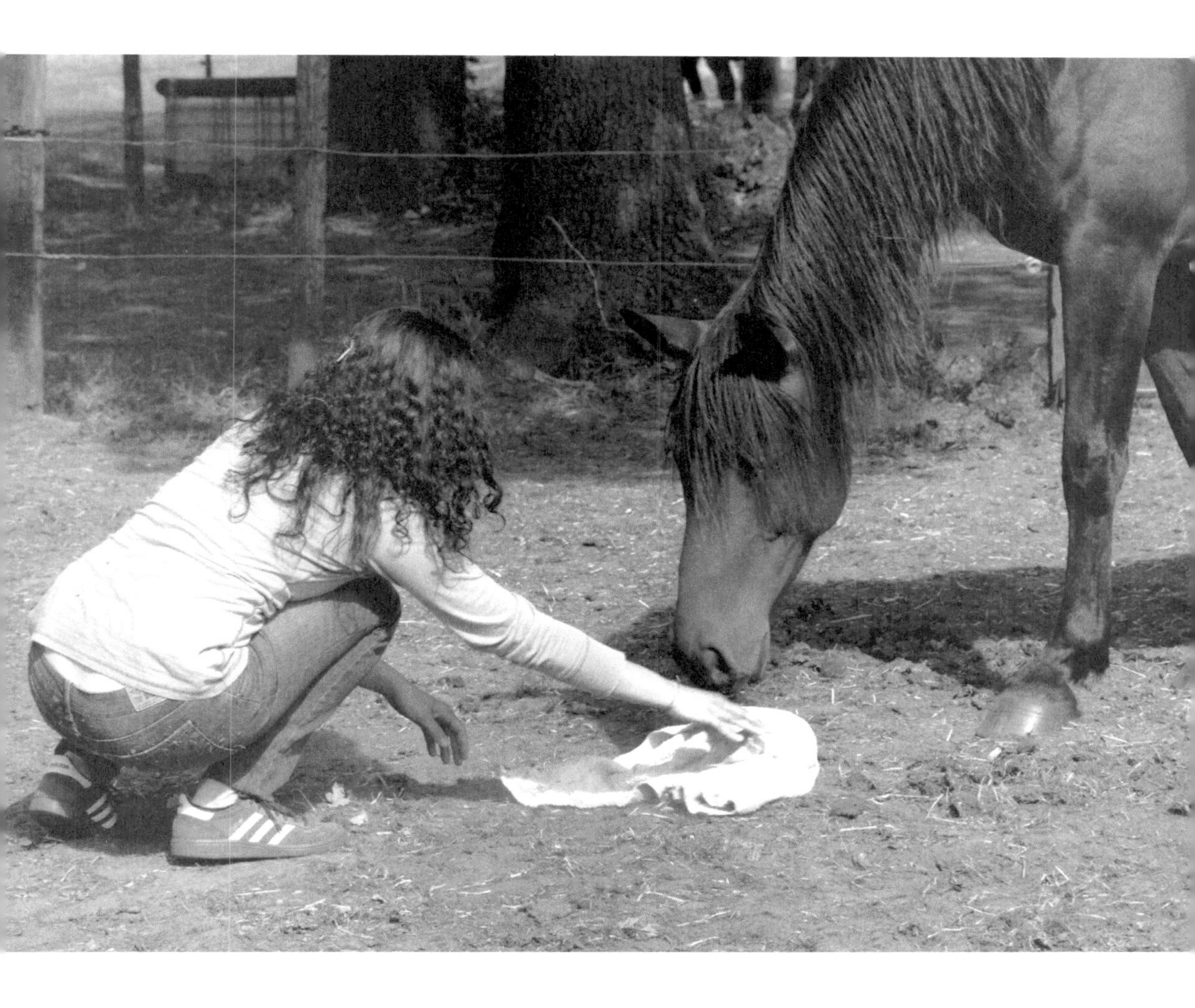

Several months and many social-learning experiences later, we arranged a short walk in the hills for Marea and her brothers and sister, accompanied by some musicians. It was one of their first experiences outside their meadow (situated in the valley), and the music created an element of continuity for them during the experience. With the sound of an accordion playing Yann Tiersen's Amélie, Marea's

eyes were soft and open, observing the surroundings and the distant views. We could sense that so much of her tension was gone and that she was enjoying the atmosphere, calmly taking in all the details of sound and nature around her.

Today, in our herd, she is one of the most curious about human contact and the sharing of experiences—a beautiful young mare who will continue to astonish humans with her fully expressed curiosity, keen observation skills, gentle approach, and pondered decision-making.

10

Applied Zooanthropology: Learning Together

From Self-Affirmation to Reciprocal Growth

For a social animal, dialogue is a fundamental element of individual growth. Both what you exchange in a dialogue and the experience itself can help you in your personal development and understanding of yourself. As the dialogue is part of a shared moment, the awareness and observation of what happens in that dialogue is very important. It is the dialogue experience that gives insight and, as such, constitutes a foundation of co-learning.

Nowadays, people tend to forget or ignore this aspect of an experience and focus instead on its result. They look at the impact of an expression or behavior on the other individual to see whether it had the desired outcome. They focus on self-affirmation and, in doing so, unconsciously train themselves to ignore all the smaller gestures and exchanges, the curiosity, and the wonder.

A typical example of this is a practice used in "leadership development" where someone stands in an area with one or more horses and is asked to see if he or she can make the horse or horses move. It is an exercise that focuses on self-affirmation and the ability or "power" to get movement out of another living being, to understand if the person can obtain a desired outcome. It is a protocol interaction, where humans only focus on the outcome (for example, whether the horse is moving or not). They seem to consider it natural for the horse to just wait for them to make him "do" something, completely ignoring the horse's social interaction.

In practice, what happens is that both the human and the horse find themselves in a reactive context, where neither knows the other, neither feels at ease, and where both have expectations. In the best cases, the horse may watch, look away, smell the ground, go to smell the human, come to stand next to him, or start looking outside the area, constantly searching for understanding and signs of affiliative behavior or possible dialogue. The human, on the other hand, for the sake of an illusionary power affirmation, pays no attention to that and simply tries to impose his presence. In the worst cases, the horse may be so caught up in the situation and the routine that he will either respond with the desired behavior or will walk away—or even flee. Thus, what the practice is really doing is preventing the possibility for a real social interaction.

Personal growth in a relationship with a horse means to become aware of yourself in your interaction with the "Other," be able to recognize the "Other's" perspective, and feel comfortable with what you are experiencing in the interaction. There is no right or wrong judgment, and there is no desired outcome or need to affirm your personal boundaries and position within a hierarchical set up.

Sometimes, for example, in a situation that is new to us, we can feel uneasy or uncomfortable; we might even feel threatened if someone (a horse) comes too close. However, if we feel uncomfortable, instead of learning yet another behavioral protocol to try to control the "Other's" behavior, pushing him away and describing it as learning how to respect our boundaries, we need to learn again that we can simply step out of a situation, even just by altering the focus of our attention. Stepping away is often perceived as some kind of weakness, but it is only the recognition of an awkward situation. Imagine yourself feeling uncomfortable surrounded by other people in an elevator; you're unlikely to push them around to prove your leadership capacity! With personal growth, the growth is in how to deal with our own attention and the attention and presence of others, to find a way of being comfortable in that situation.

It is also important not to misinterpret a horse's behavior or project our needs onto him. For instance, in the first example given above, we may be tempted to project our need for guidance onto the horse, perceiving him as being lost, while most horses are, in fact, simply looking for signs of affiliation and trying to cope, in a social way, with a context that is not their safe haven. They look for contact, not to be told what to do. If we want to learn from the horse and from our interaction with him, we must safeguard the cognitive context and experience, for the human and the horse, by working on awareness and curiosity toward the elements of the relationship dynamics.

Zooanthropology is essential in the process of bringing us back to learning from and working on relationship development. By focusing on relationship dynamics and reciprocal dialogue, horses and humans are both able to share learning experiences, without expectations, making it possible for them to expand and enrich their interaction, and thus grow together—each in their own way.

Finding the Right Context

"Growing" means being able to expand our personal boundaries without going over them, and this is possible *when* we start to work on the boundaries. More specifically, the work focuses on the border itself—the area where we feel comfortable and in contact with our own selves but are also in touch with the world around us.

In their interaction with horses, humans need to find a context in which both they and the horses feel comfortable (as both have the right to have a balanced experience).

Unfortunately, today people cross their boundaries continuously, and expect horses to do the same. People have learned so much from behavioral protocols that they have forgotten how to "be" and how to do things in contact with themselves and the world around them. They learn tricks, methods, and techniques to become "good" at something, but they do so by including many awkward moments in the process, as well. They are so used to these awkward moments that they even think they are a matter of course, but they aren't. Growing in the cognitive context does not mean abandoning your comfort zone in order to be able to do new things, as this would mean growing without being in contact. Finding ourselves outside our comfort zone would make us need to find results in order to feel confident again.

▶ *A safe haven for a foal can also be walking with an aunt, while the mother is already in the valley with the other herd companions. Understanding context is a need for young and old.*

Indeed, growing doesn't mean needing to affirm ourselves getting desired results or specific behavioral responses. Dialogue and learning can happen as long as both horse and human are consciously involved in the cognitive experience (without reactive behavior) and the relationship dynamic is calm and fluid. For example, when a young horse experiences the halter, it doesn't matter what the outcome is—it doesn't matter if the halter actually goes around his head. What matters is that the foal can create his own learning from encountering the halter. This means that the "experience" could be just the horse smelling the halter. It can be staying outside the paddock and rubbing a halter against the fence while both horse and human look at it; the horse might then come up to smell the human, and that's it. It can even be burying the halter under some sand inside the paddock. All these dynamics can be learning experiences and shared moments between horse and human. They allow the horse to elaborate an idea of the halter, and they allow us to develop a dialogue with the horse. They are not attempts to desensitize the foal with regards to the halter, nor are

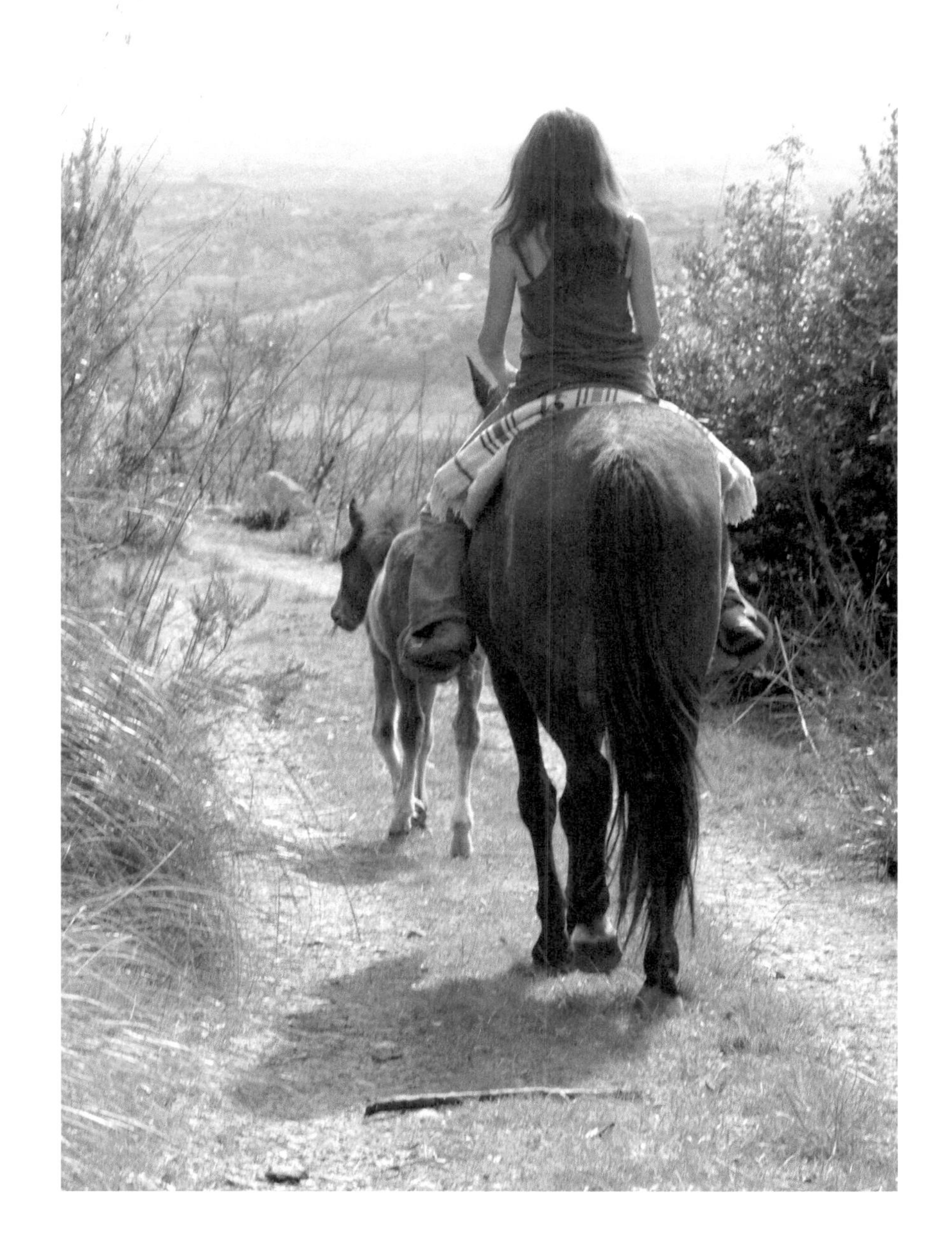

they set tasks in which the human needs to achieve a result. They are moments in which both can experience a shared world and grow from the experience itself.

If we want to share an experience with a horse, to find contact with him and create a dialogue, we must first be able to be in contact with ourselves, as only then can we explore and expand our boundaries and be able to appreciate, understand, and respect the horse's perception of a situation.

As mentioned earlier, there is no activity manual that guarantees a reciprocally interesting interaction or any set objects to use or methods to follow. For example, in the same way some people feel awkward just sitting in a meadow but don't mind checking out the fence, some horses may be curious when they see someone sitting in a meadow, while others might become suspicious or irritated but find observing a person who is checking the fence more interesting. There is no right or wrong. Every experience is unique, every situation is different, and every individual differs in what causes calm and intrigue, or closing up and resistance. We can only learn to become softer, more open, and agile in enjoying whatever experience is lived. We can learn to read the signs, be present, accept the fact that we may need to change our ideas to create room for exchange, and understand the "Other's" boundaries of being comfortable and cognitive, as well as our own.

Growing and learning how to be aware of the present moment usually requires breaking schemes because we are sometimes so conditioned that we can only focus on an expectation. This is true for both the human and the horse. For example, when we go into a field and see a horse, we often focus immediately on putting his halter on. Instead, we can break this scheme by following a different course of events and noticing, at each stage, how we (and the horse) are feeling. When you enter, just walk ahead; at a certain point, stop and drop the halter; then continue walking, away from the horse. After a couple of yards, stop to look back. How do you feel? What does the horse do? By introducing a new dynamic where automatic responses are interrupted, decision-making becomes possible. The horse can find his own inner motivation and decide whether to go to study the halter or walk toward you. Some horses might not even notice that you've dropped the halter if they are not used to taking in details anymore, so then more schemes have to be broken.

Learning to "be" is essential for personal growth and is crucial for a cognitive relationship. People tend to rush things and deny the socio-cognitive needs and expressions of a horse (especially his exploratory need in or around his living environment), and in doing so, easily create tension. It is we who provoke horses' reactions and initiate the vicious cycle: when we see their reactive state, we think we must train them in behavioral protocols, convinced that they need to be managed. The traditional anthropocentric approach exposes horses to reactive environments that cannot guarantee a quality of life. On the contrary, when the relationship is central to the horse-human interaction, there is room for growth. Understanding cognition is not a way to improve performance, but a way to learn about the quality of life.

Back to Our Senses

Creating the right learning context for a horse can be difficult at first, as we need to learn to be present without trying to direct the events or have expectations. We also need to learn to observe how he feels and behaves from his own inner world, and become intrigued by it.

For instance, we can look at a horse that is listening to something and just watch him until he turns his attention to something else, or we could try to listen, too. Even if our senses and abilities are different, it is surprising how many details we then suddenly start to hear or see. We are no longer used to really listening or observing; we have forgotten to take time and be aware of our senses.

Similarly, when a horse comes up to smell us—for example, if he smells our hair—we can choose to wait until he has finished or we can ask ourselves if we can smell or feel something, too. When we become aware of the horse's nostrils and his breath, when we become curious and also wonder how that moment "smells," we start to share the moment, instead of passively waiting. By taking part in "experiencing" the moment, we get closer to the horse, and closer to ourselves.

▶ *Learn how to wonder again, together.*

To understand relationship dynamics, allow ourselves to be curious and surprised by someone else's world of understanding, and use our senses to experience a moment, we need awareness of the following elements:

- Our focus: where does our attention go?
- Our inner state: is it calm enough to be open toward the "Other," to be able to listen, observe, and elaborate what we see?
- No dependency on a method or protocol; every relationship is unique and depends on knowledge, understanding, and awareness; every moment and interaction is situational.
- No expectations—just curiosity.

We also have to learn to do things in a new way, or rather learn again what we're no longer used to doing:

- Let go of control.
- Be patient and allow ourselves to get involved.
- Be engaged and interested; be curious toward our horses; start elaborating information by using our senses again.
- Be aware of how our focus can shift from our own perception to trying to understand what the "Other" is perceiving (even if we won't get a precise answer).

Gradually, this greater curiosity, openness, and awareness will become part of us and our daily lives, even when we're not among

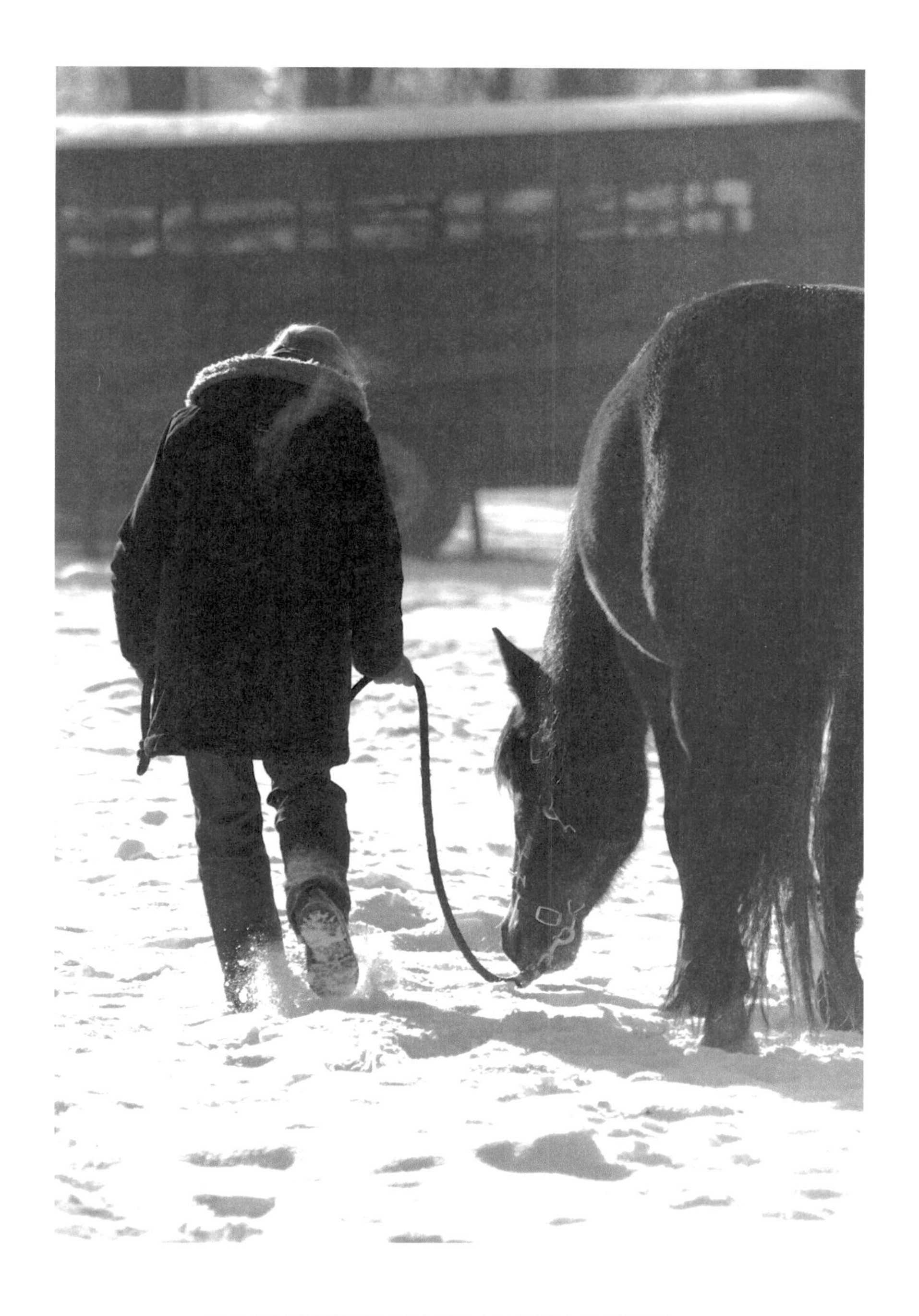

horses. For many people, it is a journey of growth. They learn about cognitive abilities, about how to preserve and respect them, and how to create room for understanding the "Other."

Cognitive abilities require a context of dialogical (characterized by dialogue) learning, where all those involved make their own cognitive heritage available, in order to build together a new knowledge and a new experience. What is important isn't the result, but how you get there, together, on a path of co-learning.

From a student of applied zooanthropology:

> *She is a beautiful young Arabian mare, but from the moment I first started working with her, I felt something was wrong. However small the steps were that I took to get her used to the saddle, or just to walk with her, I sensed that we didn't understand each other. Every initiative ended in a conflict, and our interaction was quickly becoming more and more tense. Something inside her was hardening.*
>
> *Now that I've learned about the zooanthropologic approach, about my mare's needs to explore and recognize her own intrinsic interest, and the necessity for me to have no expectations and simply allow her to explore with the rest of the herd, things have gradually changed. She now feels that she can pay attention to things without being distracted by the pressure of my tense human presence and expectations. I've started to talk differently, too: whereas I used to use a rather excited voice that kept me in some kind of trance (it was a way of keeping me in my head without really noticing what was happening around me), I now often remain silent. I am busy noticing all the smaller gestures, including my own movements, and what effect they have on the specific horse I may be approaching, as well as on the herd in general.*
>
> *I now often see her looking for experiences during the day—exploring the soil, observing the other horses, lying down, and trying to settle in the right position. We also explore things together and she has become very calm and open in our interactions. It wasn't easy to let go of my habit to control things, but it has been so worthwhile!*

11

From Performance Back to Relationship

A Performance-Oriented Society

Our society is performance-oriented. We learn to behave in the correct way to get the right "result" in social interactions. We shake someone's hand or give him a kiss even if we don't want to. We are convinced that we can "stage" a good interaction if we all agree upon the conceptual idea we create together of what a "good" interaction would look like. We perform the right macro-protocol behavior to get the picture right.

And it actually seems to work because in the process, we also get better at ignoring the nuances that are linked to smaller gestures and indications of one's emotions and inner states. We forget our own intrinsic state and motivation. Thus, if you ask someone if he's tense, it isn't uncommon for the answer to be yelled at you, "No, I'm not!" while the message is, in fact, "Please ignore the fact that I'm tense." We forget how to be curious about someone else's world of perception, about their intentions and ideas, and instead focus only on their reaction to our presence.

Yet, we have become used to this behavior, and many horses have, too. They have even become numb in the dialogue with each other as they seldom live experiences in which they can be curious toward one another, and feel in contact with themselves and comfortable enough to follow it up.

Out of the Box of Automatic Expectations

Learning how to perceive a moment starts with being curious about what that moment tells us, and for this to be possible, we have to avoid creating expectations. Expectations only fix a picture in our mind of the behavior we feel should fit a situation and make it difficult to notice other behaviors. We tend to look in linear action-reaction patterns, although there are many other elements that can color an interaction.

A friend of ours, who works as a naturalist and specializes in the study of insects, likes to go out for rides in the mountains with his young gelding. He, obviously, has a keen eye for detail, but as is often the case in the horse world, the myths, habits, and reactive environment made him feel the need to control the horse and gradually stop noticing the details of the horse's world of perception as well as the contact itself between human and horse.

As he had many questions and problems with this young horse, and the trail rides had become a continuous conflict, he came to live with us and our herd for a couple of days. We told him to watch us in our daily care and interactions with the herd. We never left the meadow. He was astonished by the amount of details we made him notice in our interactions with the horses, as well as in their interactions with each other.

Then he went back home to allow the meaning of everything he had seen (and its contrast with everything he had previously learned to ignore or take for granted) sink in. After a while, he wrote to us and told us that going out for walks had now become an adventure for both of them. When they go out, he rides a bit, then gets off to examine a particular insect and the gelding often comes over to check what he is looking at. Their going out has become a relaxed experience instead of a fight for control.

Understanding cognition also has to do with micro-behavior, noticing details, and considering even very small expressions as dialogue, because horses observe a lot in their daily lives, but don't always show obvious behavior. For instance, horses elaborate a lot of information while grazing, but if a horse observes an object that is 10 feet away for 20 minutes, we are often unaware of it, think he isn't interested, and replace the object with another we think the horse will consider more appealing (which is synonymous in our minds with something that will provoke a more visible and often reactive response). We think about how we would deal with an interesting unknown object, namely by going toward it, skipping the olfactory information and the observation of the object in its wider context. When a horse is interested, he can sometimes be satisfied with just the information he is gathering from his current perspective, even from a distance; at other times, he may also want to further his observation by getting closer, but grazing toward it, and not driven by an urge to arrive.

Similarly, a horse standing still over an object is often misinterpreted as the same as human awkwardness (not knowing what to do, experiencing a kind of blank "cloudy" moment), and the moment is consequently often interrupted. The horse might actually have been elaborating information about the object or about his inner state while standing near it.

Our expectations and projections make it impossible both to recognize such interests and elaboration processes and understand what a cognitive learning experience looks like. The more extreme approach of confronting the horse with suddenly appearing or disappearing objects and sounds in order to see his response is an unethical practice that trains the horse in reactivity and increases his state of tension, rather than allowing a calm, explorative attitude.

We can learn many things from horses, if they are free to express themselves. We can learn, for example, from their ability to observe a social dynamic in its entirety, as well as take time to decide what to explore and when. Sometimes, for a particular horse, it could even be more interesting to observe another horse interacting with an object rather than exploring the object himself, as it gives an opportunity to learn something more about the other horse.

▶ *We shall not cease from exploration*
And the end of all our exploring
Will be to arrive where we started
And know the place for the first time.
—T.S. Eliot

The less you expect, the more space remains for things to happen. The most difficult part is not how to ask, but how to experience. We don't have to learn how to ask in order to get the right answer, but how *not* to ask in order to create room for expression.

Breaking Down Schemes

Instead of thinking in terms of linearity (and action-reaction schemes), we have to think in terms of context (like the infinity-to-infinity explanation on p. 83).

Every interaction is part of a context and we need to ask ourselves, each time, what this context is. Are there other horses present? What are the dynamics between them? Is it a known environment? What is our human impact on the situation? Are we creating tension or do we have expectations?

We also need to learn to recognize and preserve the "good contexts" in which all individuals are able to use their cognitive abilities in a balanced interaction.

However, in order to do this, to start breaking schemes and automatic responses, it is essential not to have any expectations. Instead of looking out for and focusing on the behaviors we expect, we need to try

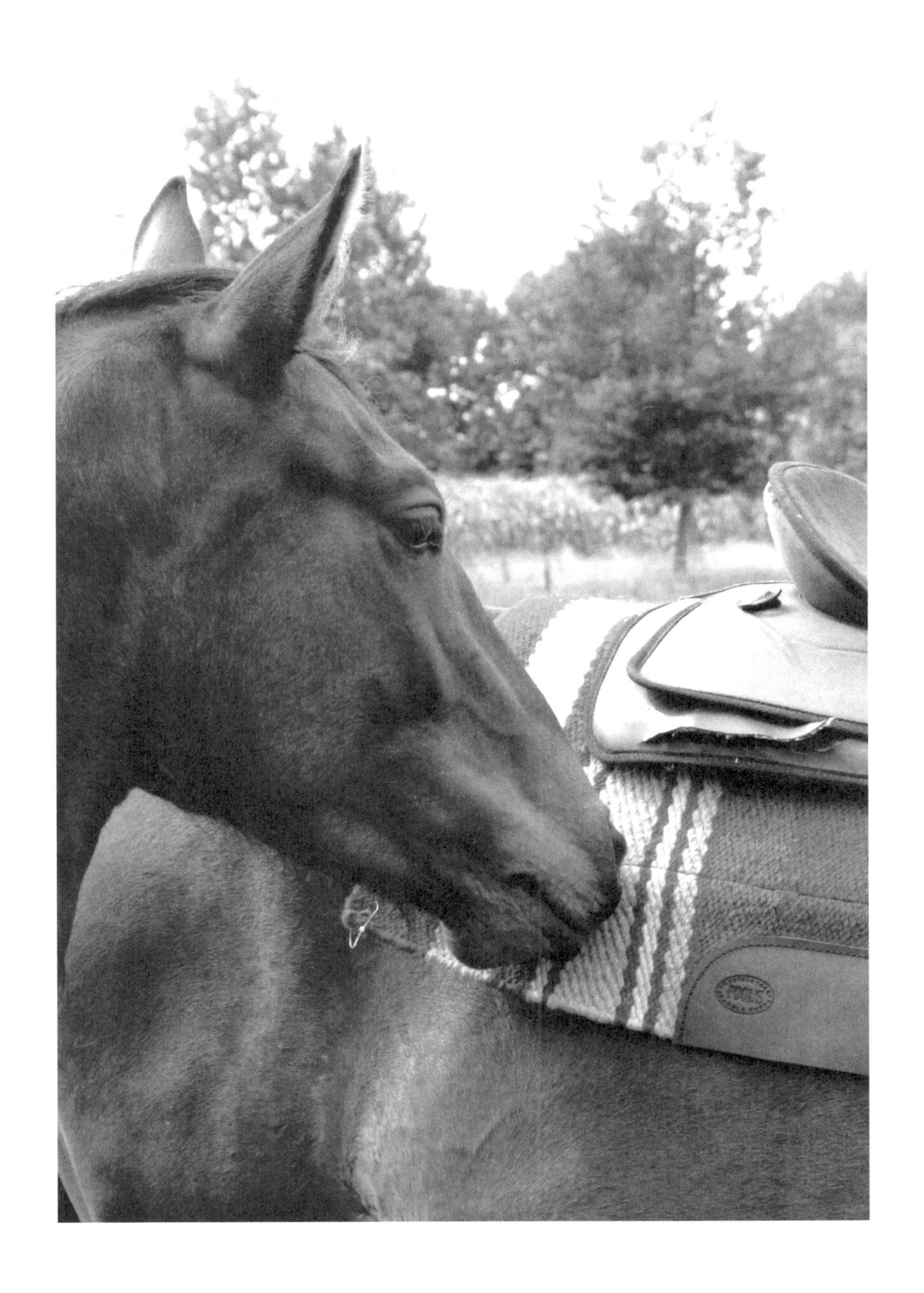

to understand what that particular horse is experiencing in that particular moment and in that particular context. Instead of focusing on the activity we had in mind, and consequently having expectations, we must be aware of the other dynamics the horse is experiencing, respect them, and take them into account.

As we become more aware of the context, this approach will completely change the focus of our own perception in a given situation, and in our interaction with horses, it will allow them to change focus, as well. It will allow the horse to rediscover the possibility of making conscious and calm decisions, and in doing so, find the value of his own subjectivity, as well as in his interactions with humans.

Here is another example of a zooanthropologic consult and how we can break schemes:

> *Lisa walked into the meadow with a yellow-colored pad. She placed it in the middle and then circled away from it to kneel down and look at it from a distance, as did Jazz, her Quarter Horse mare, who would walk away every time Lisa walked into the meadow. For a couple of minutes, it seemed as though Jazz was not interested in anything happening, but watching more closely, we could see that she had slowly turned to look both at Lisa and at the pad. After a few more minutes, we told Lisa to walk slowly toward the pad, simply taking in the intensity of its color. The moment she started walking, Jazz went toward the pad, as well. They both arrived and Lisa heard Jazz smelling, not a suspicious snort, but an intense smell, after which she turned her head to smell Lisa's shoulder and, at the same time, Lisa noticed hoof prints on the ground, the smell of the meadow, and how soft Jazz's movement had been. She walked back to the fence, leaving Jazz with a soft look in her eyes that she hadn't seen for a long time, which she felt was probably similar to her own.*

"My nine-year-old mare is a bit of a bully. She just 'walks over you' and continues to do so when you walk in her paddock."

This is a typical example of when people think they are being "tested" and of an "action-reaction mechanism" where a person, faced with what he perceives as a difficult or challenging behavior, reacts by wanting to control the horse. In fact, these problems often occur with horses that are very keen observers but no longer know how to observe when the human is around, because there never seems to be the time

Frozen Fingers

When I am with horses, I let myself be inspired by many things.
I can turn a cold Dutch wind into the wind of a timeless land.
I feel my cold-frozen fingers gently holding the reins
and I experience a jump into different dimensions, a different perception.
As in a time-machine between the horses,
among the horses, in that moment, going to past and future.
I can hear the calls of Canada geese in flight,
and now I find myself in Saskatchewan, over two centuries ago.
I leave footprints in the snow with those horses, then I find traces of bear
and feel an energetic shiver go up my back.
I feel the call of other horses and moose and wolves.
In my hair feathers of crow, hawk, and eagle appear.
I become what I have always been,
I become who I never was.
My imagination becomes a shared experience with the horses.
Together we have created our secret adventure.

and the opportunity or sufficient understanding. During a zooanthropologic consult, to allow the owner to see the horse from a different point of view, and to offer the horse the possibility to break her routine responses and find the space of a more conscious way of interacting, we worked together with the mare and her human companion in the paddock to learn to break up their habit-driven schemes. In this case, the most important element was to give the mare the necessary space and understanding that would allow her to follow her need to explore. Having the owner focus on a tree with the invitation to go and explore it from nearby, the mare, at first, looked as if surprised by this change of attention, then came closer in a calm approach and started to explore the tree as well with an intense smell. Suddenly, some people parked a car on the road and got out. The owner of the mare turned around and looked at it, with the mare turning around beside her. They stood there for several minutes, just looking together at the people arranging bags in the car—shoulder to shoulder, concentrating, and not a trace of conflict or misunderstanding.

Imagination

How can we let go of this linear tendency to control a behavioral outcome? How can we just create an experience? It requires creativity. And to encourage creativity, we need to awaken perception and make room for imagination.

By being in contact with the horse's habitat, we can create a joint journey of discovery for both the owner and the horse. It could involve discovering and exploring a branch (its rough surface, its smell, its marks of time), a beautifully colored blade of grass, a feather (an eagle's feather...a dove's?), a wheelbarrow, or a fence. The initial problems related to the "impertinent" horse tend to fade away on their own once the horse finds his way back to being curious about his surroundings. In a situation that is free from expectations and pressures, where the human is there without being there, the horse can start to open up. He can find and take the time to experience his own perceptions, he can feel the new free space around him, and he can follow his exploratory desires and needs to cognitively understand his context, his interactions, and his relationships. Imagination is crucial. It is good medicine against tunnel vision and automatisms. It represents the mutual discovery of uncharted territory.

These situations can also be created when you are still outside the paddock in order to give the horse the opportunity to observe before you enter his field and before the automatic behavioral responses start. It could involve moving something but interrupting progress and taking the time to observe what is happening, regulating your movements in ways that gives the horse time to experience his curiosity and avoid tense reactions.

Creating these situations allows new dimensions for dialogue, exchange, and sharing.

12

Co-Learning: Developing the Future

Look for Experiences, Not Results

Learning that interactions are situational and that we can live in the moment is an important start. Being "open" to the moment is also facilitated when we develop our curiosity and open ourselves to the world around us by using our senses again. Too often, we look without seeing. We recognize things with our mind without actually realizing what it is that we are seeing. We look at a horse and say, "She is watching us," without wondering what makes us think that. We also tend to look without giving our full attention, picking up only a few details and forming our conclusion from them. We forget how to be curious, although it is an important inner state that is crucial for learning and to avoid judging.

Many of the humans and animals that follow the cognitive-zooanthropological approach experience a feeling of homecoming because it conceptually and practically works to avoid the alienation caused by regulatory mechanisms. By losing their need for control, people can better understand themselves and their dialogical relationship with the horse and, as a result, can finally perceive the horse as he truly is.

"Zoomimesis" for a Richer Dialogue

When we start moving within a herd, it is important to be open to everything that might arise and to observe it with fresh eyes. Gradually, as we break the schemes we used to use to look at things, and in doing so, remove the filters that hid or colored so many details, we become aware of new dynamics. We can learn to live and experience these dynamics by changing perspective, watching from a different position, changing posture, or trying to reproduce the movements of the horses we observe.

The movements we make when we mimic the behavior of an animal are called *zoomimesis*. Mimicking enables us to become aware of certain, more subtle behaviors, like the fact that horses move in semi-circles when grazing, or take little pauses when they interact with others. As we try to keep up with the horse's movements, we begin to notice even the smallest movements and behaviors, and we start to elaborate these different details that our brain usually filters out. Zoomimesis is not about mirroring the other, which would make us focus on the result, but about gaining new insight and trying to understand how our perception changes when we empathize with the movements of someone else. Through comparison and hybridization (mixing experiences—sharing an experience and being inspired by another's perception and point of view), it enriches our operational and cognitive perceptual apparatus and facilitates dialogue.

The main elements of zoomimesis are:

- Comparison: to relate our own behavior to that of the animal "Otherness."
- Dialogue: to seek forms of complementarity (working well together) between our own movements and the animal's.
- Partnership: to build synergies in experiences.

"When man still did not have his technological equipment, the animals were his promoters of knowledge, as observing the behavior of other species meant having a key to understanding the world and consequently increase the chances of survival."
—Roberto Marchesini

In zoomimesis, the horse is no longer an object of knowledge but a partner of knowledge, which is how things were, originally.

By simply observing an animal and learning from our differences and similarities, we are able to increase our knowledge and understanding of him and of ourselves. Indeed, we can only truly learn from an interaction with an animal when what we learn comes from our own introspection, rather than from someone else providing an interpretation.

▶ *Observing you makes me listen to myself.*

Zoomimesis also makes it easier for the animal to observe humans as there is less "noise" around, and in doing so, he is driven by curiosity rather than defensive reasons.

Reciprocal Understanding

The possibility of having a reciprocal, non-anthropocentric relationship starts in a situation where both horse and human are able and free to express themselves, make calm decisions, take initiative, and choose whether or not to be involved.

When a horse walks up to us but comes too close, instead of starting "personal-space/boundary-protection attempts," we should be able to just step away. That is how socially balanced beings living in a friendly context communicate that they do not want to be involved. When someone sits down too close to you on a train, you will probably just shift away, not start making strange gestures! It is our conviction

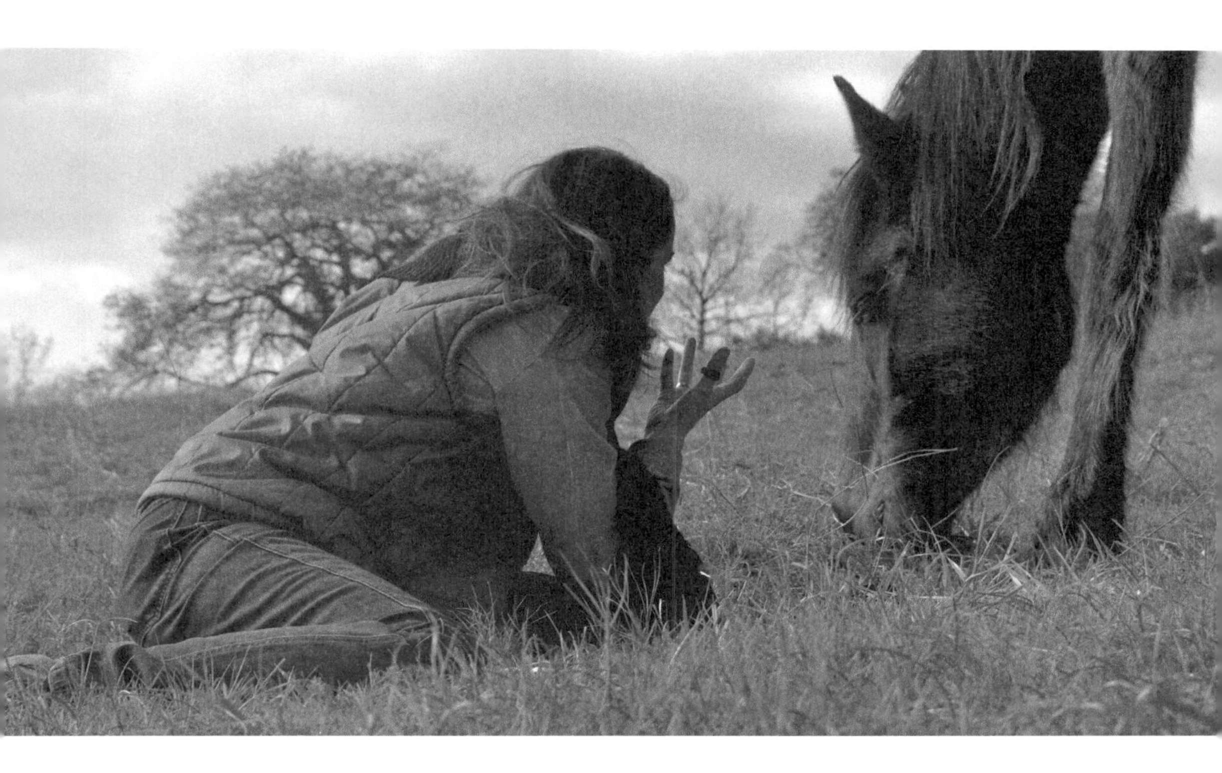

that we want to decide what to do that makes us victim to the conditioned assumption that we need to be in control. Yet, we can just step aside. In fact, it is much easier, and many people have been pleasantly surprised by how nice it is to step out of the contact, as this gives room to be curious toward the situation, instead of starting to feel defensive. And, maybe you'll find the horse simply standing there, without insisting, enjoying the standing together.

A horse will never be a human and a human will never be a horse. Yet, in the two worlds of perception they each create for themselves, there is an overlap of understanding that we can learn to recognize and develop together into a shared dialogue that belongs to that particular relationship.

This is what the zooanthropologic approach is all about. It cannot be a protocol or a method that is simply copied and pasted onto any arbitrary relationship and situation. Not only is each situation and relationship unique, but the fact of being able to share moments and enjoy each other's presence also requires both the horse and the human to be able to consciously perceive an experience.

Paradoxically, it is the conditioned horse—the horse that has been trained to perform activities with man, but hasn't been given the opportunity to listen to his own inner motivation or act freely in his

Exercises or Experiences?

What is the difference between performing an exercise or living an experience? For many, probably nothing. In this case, an exercise is defined as an experience. But there is, perhaps, something very different when seen from different points of view.

Following a classic definition of the meaning of exercise, we can identify a number of distinctive aspects: the presence of a result to be achieved, an expectation connected to that result, the pursuit of precision in the execution of the exercise, and the tendency of automatic movements to bring the execution of the exercise to a level of perfection.

If we take into account some terminology commonly associated with the word "exercise," we find the following: train, prepare, instruct, educate, teach, getting used to, drill, performance, test, discipline, workout, exertion, pursuit. This brief sequence of related words, might help us understand the kind of context that exercises impose on animals in their interactions with humans.

Now to another representation linked to the experiential dimension instead.

interactions with man—that resists, throws his rider off, runs away, avoids being caught, or becomes closed and just follows commands.

Once we develop the ability to look at socio-cognitive herd dynamics, reciprocal understanding can be extended to the entire herd, and we can discover a new world of interactions: stand next to each other, look from a distance, walk and stop, and more. A herd is a living organism where all the elements are both themselves and part of the whole (as they share the same experiences). It is like a theater in which humans can learn to take part. By working with the socio-cognitive approach,

This experience is characterized by some unambiguous very different meanings, or better, the absence of certain elements: the absence of a result to be achieved, the absence of expectations to respond to, the absence of a search for a precise execution, the lack of automatic responses.

All these absences give space to something different: space to overthrow the *interaction paradigm*—that is, how we interact with, learn from, and relate to another. Learning, being in tune through shared experience, has a great value from a socio-cognitive, emotional, and perceptive point of view.

From a sociological, ethological, neuro-physiological, and cognitive-zooanthropologic point of view, exercises on the one hand and experiences on the other, fall into two different and distinct categories, and they are do not overlap. This distinction doesn't bring a positive or negative value; they simply represent two different worlds, two different ways to approach the "Other," understand learning, understand relationships. Ultimately, they are two different approaches to living life.

All people have the option of making a choice about which dimension they want to interact and live with, as long as it is a choice based on knowledge, ethics, conscience, coherency, transparency, and clarity.

horses that have forgotten they can take each other into account and merely live as a group of separate, individual horses can learn to become a herd.

We can learn many things from a horse, but we must remember that he has his own learning path. He isn't a whiteboard on which humans can start writing. Each horse should follow his own path, and have his own, growing understanding of himself and the world around him. In fact, both the human and the horse need to follow their own path of discovery. Both need to learn to be aware of their own bodies. Both need to preserve proprioception (sensory information that contributes to the sense of position of self and movement) not impacted by bits or shoeing. Both need to become more aware of their inner states, find their own motivation, and understand how they can learn from others, and how to be grounded and emotionally balanced.

Nowadays, many people are not interested in training their horses to become soldiers or puppets, but want to know them better by understanding their real needs, work on their quality of life, and develop a true and open relationship. As the conventional language used in horse culture makes it difficult to take the horse's point of view into account, it is now appropriate to start altering this language in order to allow a real change of terminology and practice in the horse-human relationship. For example, we should consider replacing the militaristic and mechanistic word "training" (and all the anthropocentric exercises that come with it) with the word "learning." Even better, we would call it "co-learning," in recognition of the human and horse growing together, finding room for shared activities, and opening up the possibility of a true dialogue by stepping free of the suffocating conventions of the equestrian world.

Obviously, this is not easy to do as the image we have of horses is universally linked to how we can "use" the horse. A person who decides to go for a walk with her horse, on foot, simply to enjoy the possibility of walking together, will most likely be asked by those she encounters if the horse is too young, or very scared, or been injured, or whether the rider fell off, because most people cannot imagine why she wouldn't be riding, as that, in their understanding, is "what horses are for."

Learning to be curious and open toward the expression of the "Other," without losing ourselves, is fundamental for a sound social-emotional experience in a society where focus is more on performance than on relationships. Both humans and horses need time and space to be able to understand their internal motivation, instead of merely reacting to a context or adopting a desired behavior. The zoo-anthropologic approach gives a horse the opportunity to create his own mental map by using his own mental and physical capacities, in which attention, awareness, relaxation, contact, and social interaction are key words, allowing spontaneous interaction and reciprocal understanding.

A New Coexistence

By now, it is commonly accepted that animals have feelings, but their inner world and the relationship between their feelings and their behavior are still often perceived as some kind of black box where stimuli go in and behavior comes out. It is almost an evolutionary process for humans to recognize animals as sentient beings and as non-human individuals with their own complex mental activities in elaborating life.

People still struggle to recognize cognition in animals. On one hand, this is because they feel it would be anthropomorphizing the animal due to our difficulty in grasping the concept of different cognitions. On the other hand, it is because if we attribute cognition to animals (other than primates), we will have to clarify what makes humans "human," and, in particular, alter the idea of the human's exclusivity in having a cognitive brain. It requires us to accept and understand different developments of the same abilities. Our behavior toward animals should be guided by this recognition. The animals we interact with turn out to have more complex mental and emotional lives than people realized in the past, and new scientific research is constantly presenting new evidence of animals' cognitive abilities and emotions.

Therefore, for our own development, and for the beneficial wellness and further understanding of our coexistence with horses, look for the cognitive horse inside *every* horse! Allow him to enjoy a socio-cognitive life (not an anthropocentric life) as that is how he is, naturally, when he is born.

▶ *Togetherness is found in the journey.*

Horses have their own capacity and instruments to be able to experience and entertain good relationships that take the "Other" into account, including interspecies interactions with humans. But they need the appropriate environment, a preserved cognition, and an equine socio-cognitive context in which to live to be able to act upon it. It's time for us to make that possible.

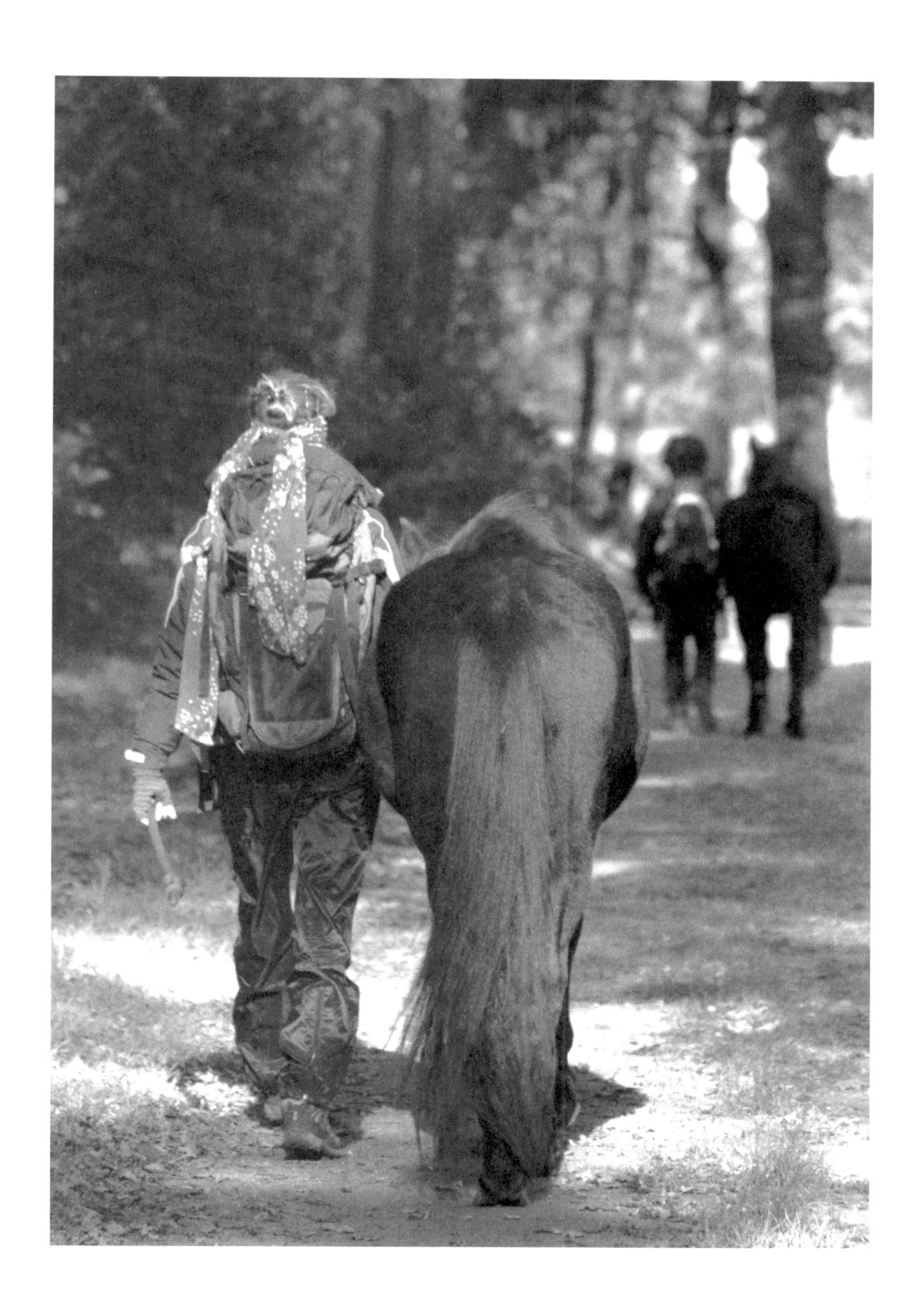

13

Beyond Horizons

A Journey Toward Ithaca

We are traveling toward a future in which cognitive ethology, the anti-speciesist philosophy, animal ethics, and a more post-human legislation regarding animal welfare will supply important change in the relationship and interaction between human and non-human animals. It is a new way of looking at our relationship with horses, which will ask horse owners, professionals, academics, animal rights organizations, and political movements to redefine decision-making processes, and break with habits and decisions that have been taken for granted for a very long time.

The ideas described in this book are part of the current cultural changes that are addressing the human-animal relationship worldwide, as speciesism (assigning different values, rights, or special consideration to individuals solely on the basis of their species membership) requires an evolution exactly as happened with racism and sexism. It is not something that will be changed overnight, but everyone can start today with curiosity toward this change—not trying to control it (either by stopping or forcing)—but resonating with it, creating new images and new activities, giving space to new insights, and building new realities together with horses and other animals.

In this process, we can find many surprises, discover how we can free ourselves from equestrian beliefs, rediscover the horse as he is, and find a relationship with him that we have always dreamed of but never had the courage to live. However, this is not magical, mystical, or paranormal, but something very concrete, practical, and sustainable both for equines and humans in their way of coexistence—free from animal training and conditioning. Rediscovering the horse is about the latest insights in animal cognition and learning, preserving him rather than training him. It is about very practical experiences—ways to live together without looking for desired behaviors, performance exercises, and anthropocentric results.

The most difficult step to make is to open new doors, letting go of the expectations of seeing what you already know, but allowing yourself to look with new eyes. Once you take that step, the journey becomes surprisingly easier and you will start traveling back home, as Ulysses did toward his beloved island, Ithaca, after he had met the Laestrygonians, a Cyclops, and the Sirens (which in our days would be represented as our own insecurities, social pressure, or traditions that are difficult to break).

It's a long journey in which you will find new lifestyles and new meanings. It brings in many aspects of questioning our way of interacting with horses, and also the other animals you may encounter during your life: sheep, cows, dogs, and cats, for example. It questions our omnivore diet, as this has everything to do with an ethical and eco-sustainable lifestyle, which is not based on a preferred coexistence with one species or another. And at the end, everyone is on a journey of development, with new insights, experiences, and adventures in life—both human and non-human animals.

How Does the Journey Start?

When you are with your horse, ask yourself these questions: How can I proceed and take these new developments in account? How can I integrate them with practical situations? How can I help the horse become owner of his own world? And what about haltering, saddling? And safety? What about activities like foot trimming and vet visits?

Oh, all these questions—but you will not find the answers without living the experience. So if you now free your mind and simply let the halter fall down on the ground, or the saddle, or the bareback pad, or the brush, the horse might be surprised by this action, but it is the first step of change in a new paradigm of relationship and interaction. Maybe the horse will approach the halter or pad on the ground to explore it, and you will do the same together with him, just sharing the moment, the experience, feeling the dust on the ground—not as a method, not to attract the horse's attention, but simply to become a human who knows how to experience his own environment.

▶ *Rediscover the horse as he is.*

To be a more natural human, seeing things with which you are already familiar with fresh eyes; considering them not for the functionality you've been taught to give them, but for what they truly are—this is something to explore, to make your own. And this means redefining the exploratory behaviors of horses that have been inhibited or desensitized by human beliefs and concepts. This means allowing that maybe we don't know how the world should look for a horse or the behavioral repertoire in which he should fit.

Start to discover them again, not as something to control, but as expressions belonging to someone's own world of understanding.

Or you could decide to stop food rewards, giving room instead to the horse's inborn motives and to the spontaneous behavior connected with them; you'll discover the space it actually gives to both you and the horse, free of expectations, and with a renewed curiosity toward each other.

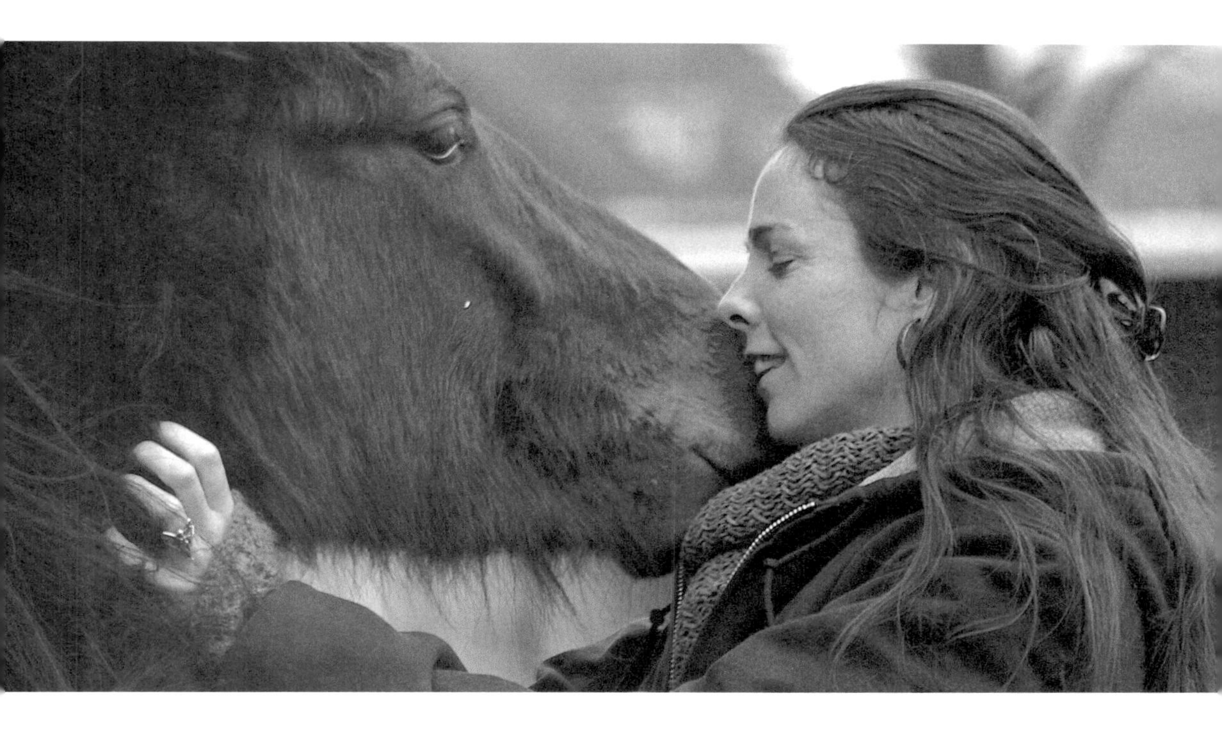

Or you might also realize that a medical treatment can become a shared experience as well. You might see a new horse with his reborn expression: emancipated and free from reinforcement. Or, you could decide to finally avoid the use of a whip or a stick. You might even discover that you are becoming curious about the smell of a hoof pick yourself, the one hanging near the shelter, which the horse just recently explored.

You are probably now thinking that these are odd things to do; maybe you are ashamed to express yourself: What will the horse make of it? What will others make of it? Do not worry. You are not alone in this new and strange dimension. It is as strange as it is liberating. Already many people have found their way back home, opening the doors to what they have always been looking for: a true dimension of interspecies relationships, where both can be themselves. It has changed their life and coexistence and interaction with other animals.

They are passionate horse people: barefoot trimmers, equine vets, acupuncturists, relationship consultants, herd facilitators, people who are revolutionizing therapy or personal growth activities, and people who work in sanctuaries. They have all learned how to develop interactions and relationships where the human is decentralized and the horse not ignored in any moment due to human desires or expectations.

We are in a society in great transformation from the animal ethics perspective, so things that looked normal yesterday will become strange today, and things that look strange today will become normal tomorrow. And in this sense, animal training that is considered normal today will become less acceptable tomorrow, as you can already see when considering that many techniques are animal abuse.

Understanding the horse as an individual does not mean finding the most humane way of training because that is still an anthropocentric view. It is about understanding an individual for who he is—for his way of experiencing and being in the world. It is about creating awareness and understanding that manipulating behavior has an impact on that individual's identity. So go on your own journey, to enrich yourself with a changing view and with new knowledge. Align it with your deepest moral values, study the frontiers of interaction with other animals, and imagine new models of coexistence with horses. The future is here.

Animal Ethics—Equine Emancipation

In recent years animal ethics has grown considerably from a minor presence in bioethics to an autonomous entity, giving back a more and more significant contribution to the field of bioethics, as well. This growth has been developed from a growing sensibility of public opinion about the arguments and issues connected with animal welfare and well-being, intertwined with animal rights, anti-speciesism, and post-humanism. Animal ethics is like a compass giving direction to a

Horses Walking in the Dust

I walk in the dust. The heat makes everything indefinite, like walking into a non-space, in a non-dimension. I put the saddle down on the ground, creating a small cloud of stirred dust.

Then, a family of horses approaches in a line. A warm breeze moves their thick, compact tails sideways, almost horizontal. Then they stop, and stretch their necks forward. Their nostrils are trying to capture the smell coming from the saddle and from me. They approach calmly; stop at times, to sniff the saddle, but without tension.

They are getting closer; I feel the sweet typical smell that originates from their skin. One of them is now near me; he approaches and explores the saddle first with his nostrils and whiskers, olfactory and tactile exploration at the same time, in slow movements. He continues to explore with his lips, sometimes stopping to exchange olfactory information with the other family companions, while their bond enriches and gets deeper and stronger in this shared new situation. One by one they join in, until all explore everything. They sniff me, too: my legs, my hair, my head, my back, my hands, the back of the saddle, with their hooves, as well, gently, a mantra-like rhythm.

Then they continue their calm walk. I see them move away east, barely visible with the dust rising up from their path.

And I wake up.

paradigm shift from an anthropocentric vision of the animal to a biocentric (considering all forms of life as having intrinsic value) one, in which everyone is protagonist of his own life inside a bigger system.

Caregivers, volunteers, and professionals who develop themselves inside the evolved framework of animal ethics will therefore have a better answer and guideline in critical situations, as well. In fact, what is right, from the perspective of an individual animal, requires a thorough understanding of subjectivity. We need to learn how to give space to the individual animal, helping him make his own decisions that fit his desires pertaining to any given situation.

▶ *Change the way you interact with your horse by not simply doing what is expected.*

Understanding this ethical perspective means that a caregiver, volunteer, or professional will put himself at the service of the horse and not at the service of the functionality of human schemes. This perspective asks to preserve the autonomy, dignity, integrity, and vulnerability of every individual horse, and in this sense, it is a process that we could call "equine emancipation": a process of animal emancipation, freed from the presumption of the horse as an instrument within the equestrian industry.

The concept of autonomy in ethics for horses is related to offering them the possibility of creating their own understanding and ideas (cognition). It is related to seeing them as moral agents and not as moral patients. It considers their right to have privacy, and the possibility of reflecting and expressing themselves without coercion or conditioning. It means ensuring the possibility of a family-like social life.

Integrity and dignity are related to understanding horses not as a particular "category" because we gave them the label of "domestic" animal. No horse is born to become a dancing object, just as bears are not born for dance performance. It doesn't matter how gentle, smooth, or how well-intended we are when we train him; it matters to further develop a common understanding of applied animal ethics.

And the last—the concept of vulnerability—is a call for humans

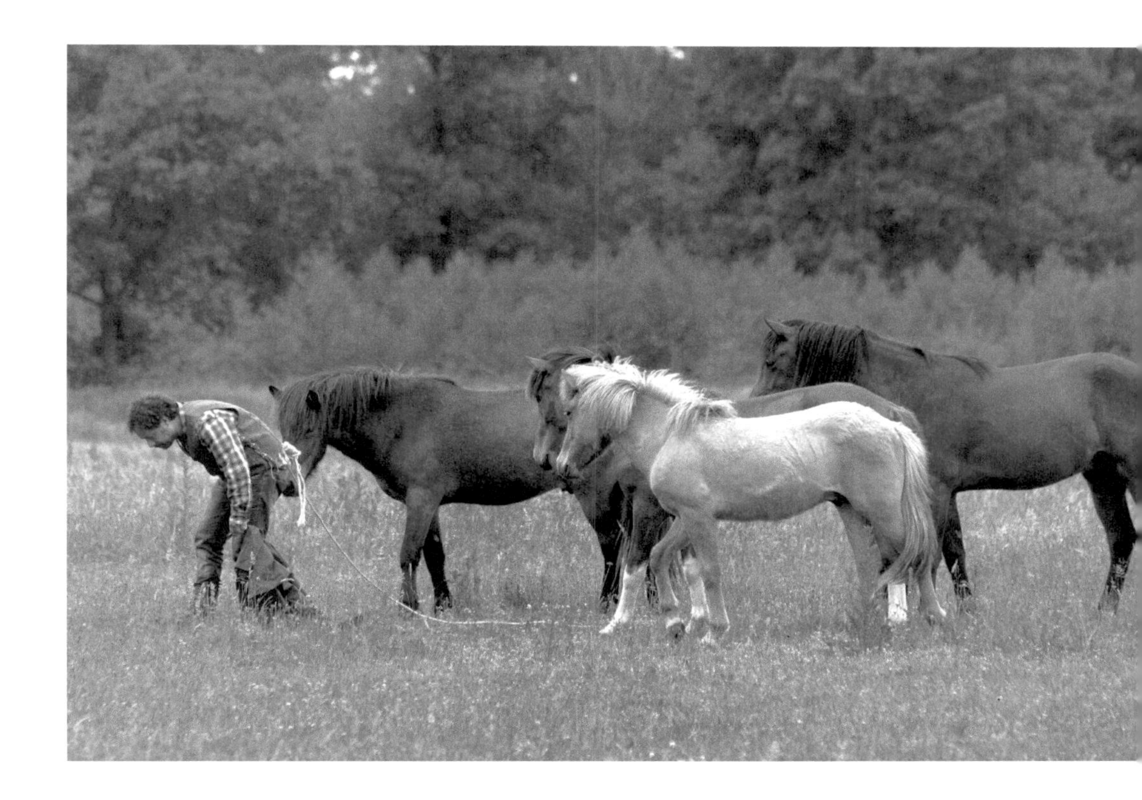

to avoid any threat to the intrinsic value and potential of an individual horse. It recognizes that this is the time to escape the heritage of exploitation interwoven with conventional habits within the equestrian industry. Equine ethics are neither boring nor utopian—but they are an opportunity to evolve and take a strong moral position when it comes to questions of our coexistence with animals.

Evolution in Professions

New professions—both challenging and inspirational—arise from this new context of equine rights, equine cognition, and equine zooanthropology. There are new surprising ways to work for the horse's quality of life and his interaction with people, according to modern animal-ethics guidelines. These ways give a refreshing view on professional development and the personal growth required.

▶ *Embrace spontaneous behavior—walk the talk.*

Animal-ethics professionals, facilitators of relationships, and quality-of-life consultants can offer a strong contribution, both cultural and professional, to further open up possibilities and create innovative fields of work in which the horse is central as a subject and an individual, and not as "instrument" or employee. But to get there it is necessary to study and learn within an ethical framework, and learn how to deconstruct the current paradigm.

Horse behavior studies and research need a different approach to avoid remaining trapped in conventional interpretations. Studying interactions free from animal training is one of the key changes, and this requires a personal growth development, as well, in which we free our own minds from conditioning shaped by social pressure, social reinforcements, and social gratifications. It needs to be a cultural change that asks professionals to have an open mind, a strong ethical preparation, and indomitable courage to break with the current schemes. It's a contribution linked to philosophical development and political activism, and even in other fields of human life. It is a global process in which all of us can choose to be a passive part or be involved as an active element for change. It is a change for humans who want to take action for other animals. It is a journey for audacious, tireless, unstoppable professionals that want to contribute to this cultural change—on every level—not just to develop their own activities but to improve equine moral status and quality of life.

Moving On

It is time to move on, not simply based on good intentions, but based on a profound development of knowledge in animal studies. Along with experience, the journey asks for curiosity, and further development of knowledge, because even if you intuitively know that a relationship

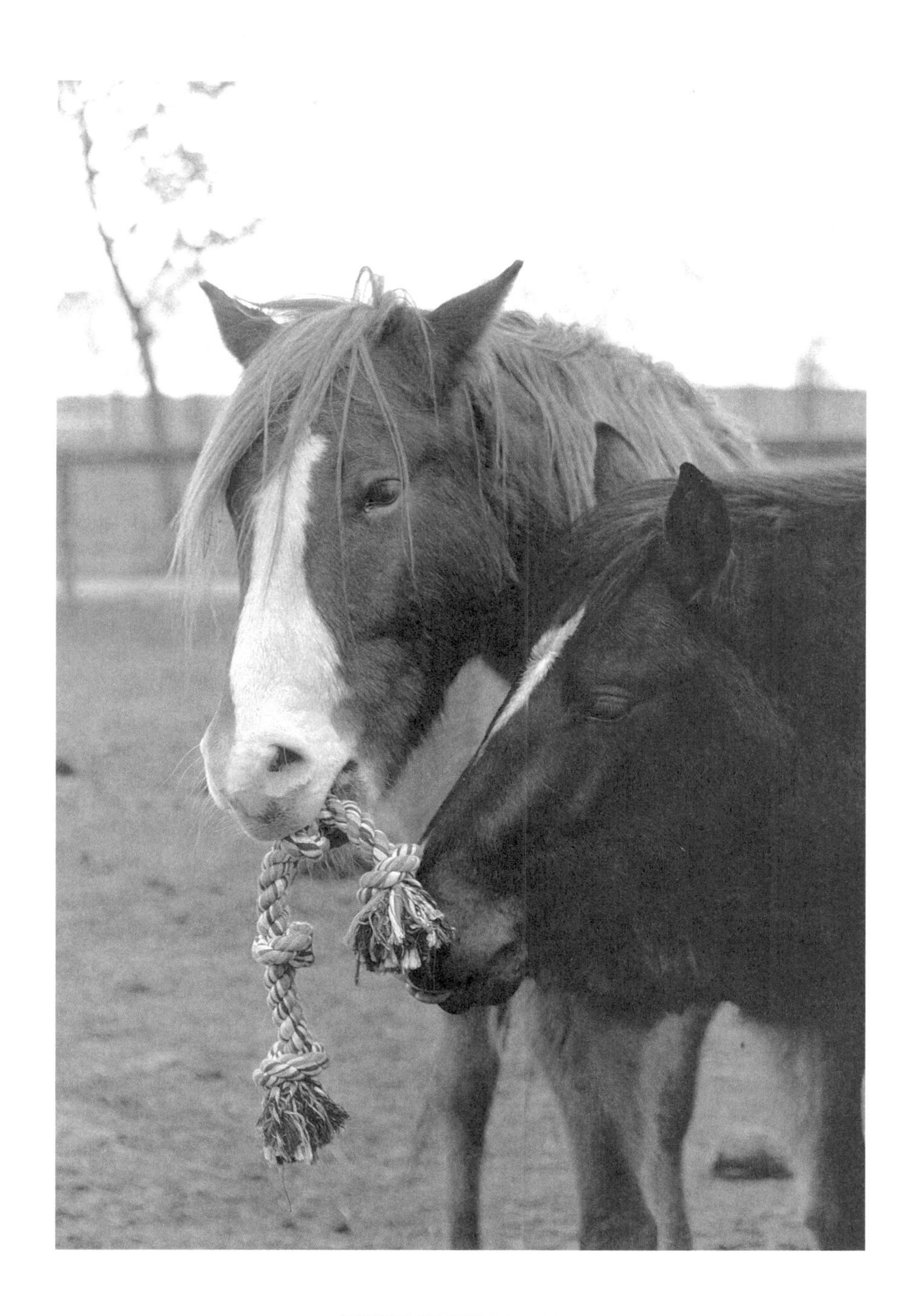

based on freedom of expression and reciprocity is the way to further develop your coexistence with the horse, you should still commit to further study in order to become aware of anthropomorphic tendencies.

These study choices are necessary, but not easy. In fact, education, both in academic or private schools and institutions, is still a mainstream education that emphasizes *old* concepts about animals, often coming from speciesistic thinking. Even programs that begin to talk about cognitive ethology and cognition can easily have a behavioristic basis that does not really understand the mental, emotional, and social life of animals but simply addresses a "bio-machine" with more sophisticated features.

Ethology has become a way to understand trained behaviors, *not* spontaneous ones. Nowadays, it is often mixed with behaviorism and equestrianism—a fatal mixture for the autonomy, integrity, dignity, and vulnerability of horses, and definitively for their (social) minds. So moving on means to study advanced and ethical references, to study cognitive ethology inside the anti-speciest and post-human perspective—a frontier education that considers horses as subjects in every moment, and applies this knowledge in daily practice in a coherent manner—that is "walk the talk." In this sense, Learning Animals, an international institute for animal studies, ethics, and zooanthropology, offers a strong ethical and innovative platform of study for caregivers, professionals, organizations, and institutions with the desire to move on toward new perspectives and possibilities in their coexistence with horses and other animals. (For more information about Learning Animals, see p. 134.)

There Were Many Horses

I have seen many horses along the riverbank. They drink, with supple body, supple neck and soft expressions.

I have seen many manes along the riverbank, light as eagle feathers, whispering with a soft breeze like leaves of a poplar.

I have seen many ears along the riverbank, listening, caressed by the wind, no tension whatsoever.

I have seen many nostrils along the riverbank, soft, open, delicate, moving gently picking up a scent, exploring, communicative.

I have seen many eyes along the riverbank, curious, open, sometimes questioning, but sweet as honey, without any shadows, without any tension, without any gloom of apathy.

I have seen many tails along the riverbank, bathed by the fresh water, following its course.

I have seen countless hooves along the riverbank, barefoot hooves, perceiving the ground and the water, sustaining vigorous bodies and minds in touch with the earth.

I have seen many humans on the riverbank, or maybe they were horses, or bison, or deer. I do not know. But they were there, proud warriors and soft and supple as the river itself.

About the Authors and Learning Animals

International Institute for Zooanthropology

About Francesco De Giorgio

Born in 1965 in Italy, Francesco De Giorgio is a forward-thinker when it comes to animal ethics, as well as a biologist, ethologist, and applied behavioral researcher. Francesco is a member of the Ethics Commitee of the ISAE (International Society of Applied Ethology), specializing in equine and canine ethology. He is also founder, developer, and facilitator at Learning Animals, a study center for ethology and zooanthropology (see p. 134), where he focuses principally on the study of animal-human interaction, ethics, animal personal growth, and rehabilitation.

Graduating from Parma University in 1989, Francesco began his career as an independent field researcher, supporting several universities while indulging his lifelong passion for horses and dogs as an Equine and Canine Learning Professional (helping owners enhance their relationships with animals). Described by the International School of Ethology (Erice, Italy) Director Danilo Mainardi as "a man who works with his head and his heart and his hands," Francesco "walks the walk and talks the talk," integrating scientific knowledge into ethical day-to-day practice. An expert in equine and canine welfare, Francesco provides expert support for institutions occupied with animal health and welfare, has served on a number of ethics committees, and acts as an advisor to courts, police, and equine rehabilitation centers in animal abuse cases and rehabilitation post-abuse.

Much sought-after as both a speaker and lecturer, Francesco presents regularly on the topic of cognitive ethology in the animal-human relationship. He also teaches at several universities and has presented to numerous conferences and symposia on ethology, cognition, and zooanthropology. This is his second book.

José De Giorgio-Schoorl

Francesco's partner in both life and work, Dutch-born José De Giorgio-Schoorl personifies the bridge between equine perception and human understanding. A shared passion for horses and keen insight in social dynamics brought Francesco and José together, and today they live in the Netherlands with their eight horse companions, four dogs, and two cats.

After many years as an adviser and personal development consultant, José is today a renowned proponent of the zooanthropological approach. As a consultant and teacher at Learning Animals, José strives to improve people's understanding of cognition and relationship dynamics, and in so doing to enhance their relationship with animals. Contending that a firm grasp of equine cognition is the vital first step to understanding horse behavior, José inspires and promotes fresh thinking via her writing and her lectures, creating effective personal growth trajectories for individuals through free interaction with horses. She has presented to conferences and symposia throughout Europe.

About Learning Animals

The mission of Learning Animals | International Institute for Zooanthropology is to emphasize concepts regarding the emotional, affiliative, and cognitive side of animals, and how to preserve or rescue it when it is impacted by previous experiences or by its necessary coexistence with humans. Learning Animals recognizes (non-human) animals as subjects and sentient beings, and applies and develops the zooanthropologic paradigm for further coexistence between human and non-human animals that goes beyond the anthropocentric point of view. It is based in the Netherlands and works on an international level to create awareness for the animal-human relationship, offering educational programs; university guest lectures; student support in research regarding socio-cognitive abilities and regarding the relationship between human and non-human animals; publishing books and articles; collaborating with animal-welfare organizations and institutions; offering consults and support; and organizing conferences, workshops, and seminars.More information can be found at www.learninganimals.com.

Abstracts

from International Scientific and Cultural Conferences

We decided to share here abstracts of some of the papers we have presented at international conferences and meetings, dealing with animal cognition, the human-animal relationship, and academic and socio-cultural developments in the field of animal rights. We are doing this because we think it important to inform you, the reader, of our tireless activity to influence thinking, even the academic vanguard, as well as to give a sense of authenticity to what we propose in this book. In the abstracts that follow, I hope you will find our message uncompromising, courageous, authentic, and innovative. We operate on many levels and in many dimensions, as we believe in connecting bridges between theory and practice, we believe in promoting the development of ethical awareness in academia and scientific research, and we believe in the most practical application of our ideas when applied to daily life as we try to develop ethical relationships in our interactions with horses.

"Is operant conditioning still an acceptable paradigm from an ethical perspective, in our coexistence with other animals?" *Minding Animals Conference, New Delhi, January 2015*

It has been many years now, that the behaviorist paradigm, both in its interpretative models and in its various forms of application (as in the case of operant conditioning), is a discussed Cartesian-like paradigm from a bio-naturalistic and cognitive point of view. Still, with the ongoing study of the human-animal relationship as an exponentially growing field of focus, and with more scientific insight and data about the emotional-cognitive side in animals, as well as the understanding of the side effects of overtraining when studying behavior in a scientific context, the trend of applying operant conditioning in day-to-day practice, focusing on stimulus-response protocols, seems to become the predominant language and approach when interacting with animals. It is even seen as a standard in certain fields—for example, in animal-assisted therapy. Operant conditioning is increasingly used in guiding pet owners and caregivers to focus on animal-obedience and as a comprehensive theory for behavior consultants, teaching which technique to apply when there is a problematic behavior. This tendency is expanded toward human animals, as well, in order to work toward a desired behavioral expression. But is it really all about the *result*? Should it instead be about behavioral *expression*? And what if these *results* lead to side effects that have an impact on animal minds? And even if there are results without apparent side effects, should we still consider it an acceptable paradigm, by a new ethical perspective? Interfering with the possibility that animals create their own dialogue with their surroundings and decide which information to find interesting? Where does it leave the animal as sentient being?

Are there alternatives to the use of operant conditioning? Some paradigm shifts are already happening in science, philosophy, and culture. Apparently it is necessary to translate these understandings into tangible possibilities and practical approaches. The translation and understanding of the paradigm shift is proposed here, explaining the impact and influence of anthropocentrism and other cultural elements, and what substituting the conditioning tendency with a more socio-cognitive approach means. This synthesis is intended to shed light on the possibility that we give value to the individuality and the socio-cognitive abilities of both human and non-human animals, and at the same time preserve the freedom for human and non-human animals to create their own world of perception in our coexistence, understanding and respecting their intrinsic value and their subjectivity.

"Moving on to a new coexistence—understanding equine socio-cognition in the horse-human relationship" *International Society for Applied Ethology Conference, Spain, July 2014*

With a growing interest and awareness for animal quality of life, and understanding of the animal-human relationship, it becomes more and more necessary to develop a practical understanding of the knowledge related to topics with an important impact on animal quality of life, as for example, affiliative behavior and cognitive abilities. This is especially the case when it comes to animals living closely in relationship with humans, and where a long history of traditions is a potential hindrance for application of new insights in both day-to-day interaction, as well as in research context—for example, regarding horses in the horse-human relationship. The principal aim of this paper is to explain the possible interference of human belief systems within applied ethology regarding horses.

Equine cognition has been shaped by the evolutionary process, both by the environmental challenges and horses' complex social dynamics, resulting in strong socio-cognitive characteristics. The understanding of these characteristics should be the foundation of any interaction with humans, starting with accepting their social needs for an affiliative environment whenever undertaking unknown interactions with humans. This means, first of all, understanding the impact of training techniques, as they might reduce the cognitive-relational abilities and disturb the behavioral expressions in the relationship with humans, as they are based on a hierarchical way of interaction. For their quality of life and an ethical interaction with humans, horses should be able to actively participate in a socio-cognitive environment, having the human as a partner in shared experiences. It means considering in day-to-day practice, the horse's socio-cognitive abilities to elaborate cognitive maps, to search for information, to process knowledge, to follow his own inner motivation, to express emotions or intentions, to solve problems, to adapt to changes, and especially, to develop relationships based on affiliative expressions. All these elements form the core of any experience, leaving behind the assumption that a horse should be trained and conditioned.

These baseline indications are reassumed in the cognitive-zooanthropologic model, where the affiliative and cognitive abilities of animals are central as they should be taken into account for the development of a reciprocal horse-human relationship that enables positive, shared experiences for both.

"Understanding equine cognition and zooanthropology in the horse-human relationship for an ethical coexistence and quality of life"
International Society for AnthroZoology Conference, Vienna, July 2014

Over the past decades, studies regarding the animal-human relationship have found an increasing audience, striving for a better understanding, positive interaction, and application in the development of activities between animal and human. At the same time, studies in equine science are yielding growing evidence and more pronounced definitions of equine welfare and well-being—for example, the importance of social learning and other cognitive abilities.

However, conventional models of interaction still create a filter that is applied to the practical understanding of equine cognition in the daily interactions between horses and humans, as the interaction protocol is still mainly based on the dominance paradigm and on an anthropocentric perspective. The result is that horse-human interaction includes training methods that facilitate an active cooperation, but seldom risks pushing to attain exactly that what one is looking for—that is, a relationship based on understanding.

A horse is a socio-cognitive animal. Equine cognition has been shaped by the evolutionary process, both by the environmental challenges and horses' complex social dynamics, resulting in strong socio-cognitive characteristics. The understanding of these characteristics should be the foundation of any interaction with humans, starting with accepting their social need for an affiliative environment whenever undertaking unknown interactions with them. This means, first of all, avoiding any kind of stereotypical impact from training techniques, as they might reduce the cognitive-relational abilities and disturb the behavioral expressions in a horse's relationship with humans.

Due to tradition and culture and our performance-oriented society, it is both difficult to accept and to apply a socio-cognitive approach, where the relationship is not based on the horse as a subordinate or object and where the focus is not on immediate results. Preserving and taking the cognitive skills into account plays an important role in avoiding tension, both in the horse and in the human-horse interaction. It means considering the horse's abilities to think, to search for information, to elaborate and process information, to follow his own inner motivation, to express emotions or intentions, to solve problems, to adapt to changes, and especially, to develop relationships based on affiliative expressions. All these elements form the core of any experience, and each one constitutes an experience by itself, leaving far behind the assumption that a horse should be trained and conditioned.

In short, for their well-being and an ethical interaction with humans, horses should be able to actively participate in a socio-cognitive environment, taking initiative from their own inner motivation and express explorative and affiliative behavior, and simply having the human as a partner in shared experiences.

These baseline indications are reassumed in the cognitive-zooanthropologic model, where the cognitive abilities of animals are central. It allows us to see and understand animals as "Others," as subjects, as differently cognitive and therefore able to provide a referential contribution. In the development of a reciprocal relationship and a socio-cognitive context where horses live and share experiences together, the focus is on the horse's abilities to build (latent) learning experiences himself, which will create a rich living environment for the horse, both with others and in relationship with humans.

Equine zooanthropology focuses on the ability to define the elements of a sound relationship between horses and humans, the definition of a cognitive context, and the ability to create awareness, inviting research to extend focus on different elements of relationship dynamics and well-being indicators.

"The Spontaneous Horse: Understanding How to Look at the Horse without Expectations" *First published in* **Relations**, *June 2014, www.ledonline.it/Relations*

As horses are often seen as anxious, unpredictable animals, the fear to let them express themselves because we are convinced that this might be dangerous and they might hurt themselves or humans involved, actually *makes* them anxious and unpredictable animals. Thus we have a strange, vicious circle. For example, the fear of being bitten by horses makes us push away their heads every time they try to understand us by smelling us or exploring us with their lips. The pushing away (or even harsher actions) transforms that intention for understanding into a tense situation of *mis*understanding from the horse's point of view.

For the same reason, we often deny them their natural social behavior. In our society, horses live too often in social isolation so they can't express themselves through social behavior, and this is something that by now we all know isn't ideal (even if most horses continue to live that way). They learn to live a life in which they wait for human commands, forgetting that they have their own true intention and unique interests. But even when they live with other horses, the groups are often not permanent, not family nor family-like. With constant changing dynamics in the group, their interaction is often focused on defensive behavior, instead of finding trust in their herd companions to express themselves in their natural cognitive way—for example, by showing affiliative behavior, moving as a herd, taking each other into account in a proactive way.

What humans often see are reactive behaviors—for example, dominance/leadership dynamics—which in family or family-like groups actually happen only in rare cases, not in random, daily routine. Social behaviors are subtle, small gestures, and often barely visible behaviors that have an important cohesive function for a herd. It is much more then mutual grooming, which is an expression that can also be part of an attempt to reduce tension. It is, for example, observing each other and the herd dynamics, looking from a distance while eating grass, pre-conflict behavior to avoid tension, and smelling each other to better understand a certain situation.

Another very important group of spontaneous behaviors is investigative/ explorative behavior, fundamental for the correct development of cognitive functions. In fact, people often use techniques, methods, and tools that deprive the horse of the opportunity to explore his reference context, other horses, the human, and himself. For example, we may ask the horse to pay attention to us instead of exploring with the intent to understand the situation the horse is in. Also, some grooming techniques, such as clipping the horse's *vibrissae* (whiskers), deprive the horse of the means to explore in appropriate ways, as they are important sensory receptors. This induces stress factors while at the same time reducing welfare.

Spontaneous behaviors are important for the horse in order to develop a cognitive dialogue. Horses that are used to reactive/defensive behavior (often in conjunction with the suppression of spontaneous behaviors) show tension in their behavior, even in very small gestures, and give us, the human, a tense feeling, although this is a feeling we are not always aware of in a conscious way. The reduction of the spontaneous behavior often happens during the initial training of young horses. In these moments horses learn to reduce their natural spontaneous behaviors to improve behavior functional for human anthropocentric desires. Operant conditioning applied during these moments (with negative or positive reinforcement) drastically reduces spontaneous behaviors, and with that reduces equine welfare. The reactive behaviors that are trained instead are too often mistaken for free-choice behavior in the human interaction. For example, running to a person in a paddock with expectation of a food reward is not a free choice. Following a human being in command-based behaviors are not free choices. The horse displays macro behaviors that please us from an anthropocentric point of view, but at the same time shows micro signals of internal conflict.

Working on and being aware of an authentic relationship is very important to further develop relationship and facilitator skills, so people can pursue a pure and sound interaction with horses. In the zooanthropologic approach, especially when working as a facilitator in the horse-human interaction, it is fundamental to give the horse the option to explore his own world and engage in spontaneous behavior. When we, as humans, pay attention to the horse and create room for his expressiveness, we start an inter-species relationship. Learning to be curious and open toward the expression of the other without losing yourself, beginning to understand how to become agile in connecting to the world and connecting with yourself, is fundamental for sound social-emotional experiences in a society where focus is more on performance then on relationships. Both human and horse should have to room to understand their internal motivation, rather than responding with desired behavior from the context we are living in.

In a different way, Learning Animals explains how the zooanthropologic approach gives horses the opportunity to create their own mental map as a social map, learning map, and human-horse relationship map. It allows them to use their own mental and physical capacities, without being conditioned, as behavior is an expression of a state of mind and not the result of direct automatic external or internal stimuli. Attention, awareness, relaxation, contact, and social interaction are key words in a spontaneous interaction.

Selected Bibliography

and Further Reading

Aureli, F., De Waal, F., *Natural Conflict Resolution*. Berkeley: University of California Press, 2000.

Baer, K.L., Potter, G.D., Friend, T.H., Beaver, B.V., "Observation effects on learning in horses." *Applied Animal Ethology.* 11, 123–129, 1983.

Balda, R.P., Pepperberg, I.M., Kamil, A.C., *Animal Cognition in Nature*. Academic Press, 1998.

Baker, A.E.M., Crawford, B.H., "Observational learning in horses." *Applied Animal Behavior Science.* 15, 7–13, 1986.

Baragli, P., Mariti, C., De Giorgio, F., Petri, L., Sighieri, C., "Does attention make the difference? Horses' response to human stimulus after 2 different training strategies." *Journal of Veterinary Behavior,* 2011.

Baragli, P., Vitale, V., Paoletti, E., Sighieri, C., Reddon, A.R., "Detour behavior in horses *(Equus caballus)*." *Journal of Ethology,* 2012.

Bekoff, M., *Social Play: Structure, Function and the Evolution of a Cooperative Social Behavior.* Garland, 1978.

Bekoff, M., "Cognitive ethology, vigilance, information gathering, and representation: Who might know what and why?" *Behavioral Processes.* 35, 225–237, 1995.

Bekoff, M., Allen, C., *Species of Mind: The Philosophy and Biology of Cognitive Ethology.* MIT Press, 1997.

Benjafield, J.G., *Cognition.* Oxford University Press, 2006.

Bono, G., De Mori, B., *Il Confine Superabile. Animali e Qualità della Vita.* Carocci ed, 2011.

Castricano, J., *Animal Subjects: An Ethical Reader in a Posthuman World.* Wilfrid Laurier University Press, 2008.

Clarke, J.V., Nicol, C.J., Jones, R., McGreevy, P.D., "Effects of observational learning on food selection in horses." *Applied Animal Behavior Science.* 50, 177–184, 1996.

Clutton-Brock, J., *Domesticated animals, from early times.* British Museum of Natural History, 1981.

Damasio, A.R., *Descartes' Error.* Penguin Books, 1994.

Darwin, C., *The Expression of the Emotions in Man and Animals.* John Murray, 1872.

De Giorgio, F., *Dizionario bilingue Italiano/Cavallo—Cavallo/ Italiano.* Sonda Editore, 2002.

De Giorgio F., Schoorl J., "Why isolate during training? Social learning and social cognition applied as training approach for young horses *(Equus caballus).*" *Proceedings International Equine Science Meeting,* 2012.

De Giorgio F., Schoorl J., Saviani G., Palandri L., Tonarelli E. "Equine social cognition; differences in the social exploratory process comparing free-roaming and domestic horses." *Proceedings Winter Meeting "Cognition in the Wild," Association for the Study of Animal Behavior,* 2012.

Devenport, J.A. Patterson, M.R., Devenport, L.D., "Dynamic averaging and foraging decisions in horses *(Equus caballus).*" *Journal of Comparative Psychology.* 119, 352–358, 2005.

De Waal, F., *The Age of Empathy: Nature's Lessons for a Kinder Society.* Three Rivers Press, 2010.

De Waal, F., Ferrari, P.F., *The Primate Mind: Built to Connect with Other Minds.* Harvard University Press, 2012.

Donaldson, S., Kymlicka, W., *Zoopolis: A Political Theory of Animal Rights.* Oxford University Press, 2011.

Galef , B.G., "Imitation in animals: history, definition and interpretation of data from the psychological laboratory." In Zentall T.R. and Galef B.G. (Eds.), *Social Learning: Psychological and Biological Perspectives.* pp. 3–28. Erlbaum, Hillsdale, NJ, 1988.

Goodall, J., Berman, P., *Reason of Hope: A Spiritual Journey.* Grand Central Publishing, 2000.

Gould, J.L., *Ethology: The Mechanisms and the Evolution of the Behavior.* W.W. Norton, 1982.

Gould, S.J., *Wonderful Life. The Burgess Shale and The Nature of History.* W.W. Norton, 1989.

Grandin, T., Johnson, C. *Animals Make Us Human: Creating the Best Life for Animals.* Houghton-Mifflin Harcourt, 2010.

Griffin, D.R. *Animal Minds: Beyond Cognition to Consciousness.* University of Chicago Press, 2001.

Hausberger, M., Roche H., Henry S., Visser E.K., "A review of the human-horse relationship." *Applied Animal Behavior Science.* 109, 1–24, 2008.

Hare, B., Call, J., Agnetta, B., Tomasello, M., "Chimpanzees know what conspecifics do and do not see." *Animal Behavior.* 59, 771–758, 2000.

Hare, B., Call, J., Tomasello, M., "Do chimpanzees know what conspecifics know?" *Animal Behavior.* 61, 139–151, 2001.

Heyes, C.M., "Social learning in animals: categories and mechanisms." *Biology Review.* 69, 207–231, 1994.

Heitor, F., Oom, M.M., Vicente, L., "Social relationships in a herd of Sorraia horses. Part I. Correlates of social dominance and contexts of aggression." *Behavioral Processes*. 73, 170–177, 2006.

Heitor, F., Oom, M.M., Vicente, L., "Social relationships in a herd of Sorraia horses. Part II. Factors affecting affiliative relationships and sexual behaviors." *Behavioral Processes*. 73, 231–239, 2006.

Jackson J., *Horse Owners Guide to Natural Hoof Care*. Star Ridge Publications, 2002.

Kiley-Worthington, M., "Cooperation & Competition—A Detailed Study of Communication and Social Organization in a Small Group of Horses at Pasture." *Eco Research Centre Pub.* 21, 1997.

Kiley-Worthington, M., "A comparative study of equine and elephant mental attributes leading to an acceptance of their subjectivity and consciousness." *Journal of Consciousness*, vol. 2, num. 1, 2011.

Krueger, K., "Behavior of horses in the 'Round pen technique.'" *Applied Animal Behavior Science,* 2006.

Laland, N.K., "Social learning strategies." *Learning & Behavior*. 32 (1), 4–14, 2004.

Le Doux, J. *The Emotional Brain: The Mysterious Underpinnings of Emotional Life.* Simon & Schuster, 1998.

Lovari, S., *Etologia di Campagna.* Universale Scientifica Boringhieri, 1980.

Mainardi, D., *La Scelta Sessuale.* Universale Scientifica Boringhieri, 1975.

Mainardi, D., *Dizionario di Etologia.* Einaudi ed, 1992.

Mainardi, D., *Nella Mente degli.* Animali ed, 2006.

Manning, A., "On the Origins of Behavior." *New Scientist,* 1996.

Marchesini, R. *Il Concetto di Soglia*. Theoria ed, 1996.

Marchesini, R., *Post-Human.* Bollati Boringhieri, 2002.

Marchesini, R., *Fondamenti di Zooantropologia.* Alberto Perdisa Editore, 2005.

Marchesini, R., *Modelli Cognitivi e Comportamento Animale.* Eva ed, 2011.

Mariti C., Baragli P., De Giorgio F., Gazzano A., Basile C., Sighieri C. "Influence of training methods on horse behavior." *VII Italian Veterinary Physiology Conference,* 2007.

Mech, D.L., "Whatever Happened to the Term Alpha Wolf?" Wolf.org, 2008.

Murphy, J., Arkins, S., "Equine Learning Behavior." *Behavioral Processes,* 2006.

Nicol, C.J., "Farm animal cognition." *Journal of Animal Science.* 62, 375–391, 1996.

Nicol, C J., "Equine learning: progress and suggestions for future research." *Applied Animal Behavioral Science.* 78, 193–208, 2002.

Proops, L., McComb, K., "Cross-model individual recognition in domestic horse *(Equus caballus)* extends to familiar humans." *Proceedings of the Royal Society B,* 2012.

Radford, A.N., "Preparing for battle? Potential intergroup conflict promotes current intragroup affiliation." *Biology Letters,* 2010.

Reed, P., Skiera , F., Adams, L., Heyes, C.M., "Effects of isolation rearing and mirror exposure on social and asocial discrimination performance." *Learning and Motivation.* 27, 113–129, 1996.

Regan, T., *Empty Cages: Facing the Challenge of Animal Rights.* Rowman and Littlefield, 2004.

Rivera, E., Benjamin, S., Nielsen, B., Shelle, J. & Zanella, A. J. "Behavioral and physiological responses of horses to initial training: the comparison between pastured versus stalled horses." *Applied Animal Behavioral Science.* 78, 235–252, 2002.

Rizzolatti, G., Sinigaglia, C. *Mirrors in the Brain: How Our Minds Share Actions, Emotions, and Experience.* Oxford University Press, 2008.

Rollin, B.E., *The Unheeded Cry: Animal Consciousness, Animal Pain and Science.* Wiley Publishing, 1998.

Rollin, B.E., *Science and Ethics.* Cambridge University Press, 2006.

Sax, B. *Animals in the Third Reich.* Continuum Books, 2000.

Shepard, P., *The Others: How Animals Made Us Human.* Island Press, 1995.

Shepard, P., *Coming Home to the Pleistocene.* Island Press / Shearwater Books, 2004.

Shettleworth, S.J., "Animal cognition and animal behavior." *Animal Behavior.* 61, 277–286, 2001.

Singer, P. *Animal Liberation.* Ecco Press, 2001.

Sondergaard, E., Ladewig, J., "Group housing exerts a positive effect on the behavior of young horses during training." *Applied Animal Behavior Science.* 87, 105–118, 2004.

Swedell, L., "Affiliation Among Females in Wild Hamadryas Baboons." *International Journal of Primatology,* 2002.

Vygotskij, L.S., *Mind in Society.* Harvard University Press, 1978.

Waran, N., Casey, R., "Horse training in the domestic horse: the origins, development and management of its behavior." D.S. Mills and S.M. Mc Donnell (Ed.), Cambridge University Press, pp. 184–195, 2005.

Wolfe, C. *Animal Rites: American Culture, the Discourse of Species, and Posthumanist Theory.* University Of Chicago Press, 2003.

Wolfe, C. *Zoontologies: The Question of the Animal.* University of Minnesota Press, 2003.

Wolfe, C. *What is Posthumanism?* University of Minnesota Press, 2009.

Index